The World H

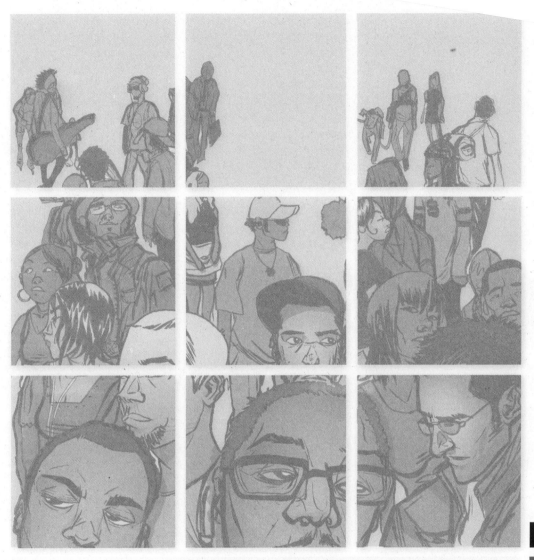

HEALTH SYSTEMS FINANCING
The path to universal coverage

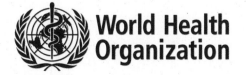

World Health
Organization

WHO Library Cataloguing-in-Publication Data

The world health report: health systems financing: the path to universal coverage.

1.World health - trends. 2.Delivery of health care - economics. 3.Financing, Health. 4.Health services accessibility. 5.Cost of illness. I.World Health Organization.

ISBN 978 92 4 156402 1   (NLM classification: W 84.6)
ISBN 978 92 4 068480 5 (electronic version)
ISSN 1020-3311

© World Health Organization 2010

This world health report was produced under the overall direction of Carissa Etienne, Assistant Director-General, Health Systems and Services and Anarfi Asamoa-Baah, Deputy Director General. The principal writers of the report were David B Evans, Riku Elovainio and Gary Humphreys; with inputs from Daniel Chisholm, Joseph Kutzin, Sarah Russell, Priyanka Saksena and Ke Xu.

Contributions in the form of boxes or analysis were provided by: Ole Doetinchem, Adelio Fernandes Antunes, Justine Hsu, Chandika K Indikadahena, Jeremy Lauer, Nathalie van de Maele, Belgacem Sabri, Hossein Salehi, Xenia Scheil-Adlung (ILO) and Karin Stenberg.

Suggestions and comments were received from Regional Directors, Assistant Directors-General and their staff.

Analysis, data and reviews of the outline, various drafts or specific sections were provided by (in addition to the people named above): Dele Abegunde, Michael Adelhardt, Hector Arreola, Guitelle Baghdadi-Sabeti, Dina Balabanova, Dorjsuren Bayarsaikhan, Peter Berman, Melanie Bertram, Michael Borowitz, Reinhard Busse, Alexandra Cameron, Guy Carrin, Andrew Cassels, Eleonora Cavagnero, Witaya Chadbunchachai, John Connell, David de Ferranti, Don de Savigny, Varatharajan Durairaj, Bob Emrey, Tamás Evetovits, Josep Figueras, Emma Fitzpatrick, Julio Frenk, Daniela Fuhr, Ramiro Guerrero, Patricia Hernandez Pena, Hans V Hogerzeil, Kathleen Holloway, Melitta Jakab, Elke Jakubowski, Christopher James, Mira Johri, Matthew Jowett, Joses Kirigia, Felicia Knaul, Richard Laing, Nora Markova, Awad Mataria, Inke Mathauer, Don Matheson, Anne Mills, Eduardo Missoni, Laurent Musango, Helena Nygren-Krug, Ariel Pablos-Mendez, Anne-Marie Perucic, Claudia Pescetto, Jean Perrot, Alexander Preker, Magdalena Rathe, Dag Rekve, Ritu Sadana, Rocio Saenz, Thomas Shakespeare, Ian Smith, Peter C Smith, Alaka Singh, Ruben Suarez Berenguela, Tessa Tan-Torres Edejer, Richard Scheffler, Viroj Tangcharoensathien, Fabrizio Tediosi, Sarah Thomson, Ewout van Ginneken, Cornelis van Mosseveld and Julia Watson.

The writing of the report was informed by many individuals from various institutions who provided Background Papers; these Background Papers can be found at http://www.who.int/healthsystems/topics/financing/healthreport/whr_background/en

Michael Reid copy-edited the report, Gaël Kernen produced figures and Evelyn Omukubi provided valuable secretarial and administrative support. Design and layout was done by Sophie Guetaneh Aguettant and Cristina Ortiz. Illustration by Edel Tripp (http://edeltripp.daportfolio.com).

Financial support from the Rockefeller Foundation, United States for International Development (USAID) and the Federal Ministry of Health, Germany, is gratefully acknowledged.

Printed in Switzerland on FSC-certified, 100% recycled paper.

Contents

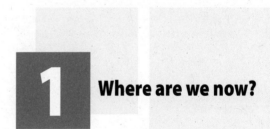

1 Where are we now?

2   More money for health

3   Strength in numbers

4 More health for the money

5 An agenda for action

103 Index

Message from the Director-General

I commissioned this world health report in response to a need, expressed by rich and poor countries alike, for practical guidance on ways to finance health care. The objective was to transform the evidence, gathered from studies in a diversity of settings, into a menu of options for raising sufficient resources and removing financial barriers to access, especially for the poor. As indicated by the subtitle, the emphasis is firmly placed on moving towards universal coverage, a goal currently at the centre of debates about health service provision.

The need for guidance in this area has become all the more pressing at a time characterized by both economic downturn and rising health-care costs, as populations age, chronic diseases increase, and new and more expensive treatments become available. As this report rightly notes, growing public demand for access to high-quality, affordable care further increases the political pressure to make wise policy choices.

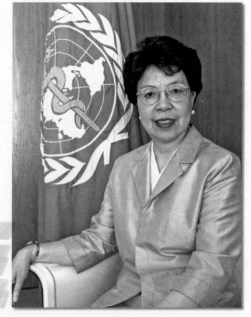

At a time when money is tight, my advice to countries is this: before looking for places to cut spending on health care, look first for opportunities to improve efficiency. All health systems, everywhere, could make better use of resources, whether through better procurement practices, broader use of generic products, better incentives for providers, or streamlined financing and administrative procedures.

This report estimates that from 20% to 40% of all health spending is currently wasted through inefficiency, and points to 10 specific areas where better policies and practices could increase the impact of expenditures, sometimes dramatically. Investing these resources more wisely can help countries move much closer to universal coverage without increasing spending.

Concerning the path to universal coverage, the report identifies continued reliance on direct payments, including user fees, as by far the greatest obstacle to progress. Abundant evidence shows that raising funds through required prepayment is the most efficient and equitable base for increasing population coverage. In effect, such mechanisms mean that the rich subsidize the poor, and the healthy subsidize the sick. Experience shows this approach works best when prepayment comes from a large number of people, with subsequent pooling of funds to cover everyone's health-care costs.

No one in need of health care, whether curative or preventive, should risk financial ruin as a result.

As the evidence shows, countries do need stable and sufficient funds for health, but national wealth is not a prerequisite for moving closer to universal coverage. Countries with similar levels of health expenditure achieve strikingly different health outcomes from their investments. Policy decisions help explain much of this difference.

At the same time, no single mix of policy options will work well in every setting. As the report cautions, any effective strategy for health financing needs to be home-grown. Health systems are complex adaptive systems, and their different components can interact in unexpected ways. By covering failures and setbacks as well as successes, the report helps countries anticipate unwelcome surprises and avoid them. Trade-offs are inevitable, and decisions will need to strike the right balance between the proportion of the population covered, the range of services included, and the costs to be covered.

Yet despite these and other warnings, the overarching message is one of optimism. All countries, at all stages of development, can take immediate steps to move towards universal coverage and to maintain their achievements. Countries that adopt the right policies can achieve vastly improved service coverage and protection against financial risk for any given level of expenditure. It is my sincere wish that the practical experiences and advice set out in this report will guide policy-makers in the right direction. Striving for universal coverage is an admirable goal, and a feasible one – everywhere.

Dr Margaret Chan
Director-General
World Health Organization

Executive summary

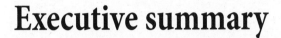

Why universal coverage?

Promoting and protecting health is essential to human welfare and sustained economic and social development. This was recognized more than 30 years ago by the Alma-Ata Declaration signatories, who noted that Health for All would contribute both to a better quality of life and also to global peace and security.

Not surprisingly, people also rate health one of their highest priorities, in most countries behind only economic concerns, such as unemployment, low wages and a high cost of living (1, 2). As a result, health frequently becomes a political issue as governments try to meet peoples' expectations.

There are many ways to promote and sustain health. Some lie outside the confines of the health sector. The "circumstances in which people grow, live, work, and age" strongly influence how people live and die (3). Education, housing, food and employment all impact on health. Redressing inequalities in these will reduce inequalities in health.

But timely access to health services[a] – a mix of promotion, prevention, treatment and rehabilitation – is also critical. This cannot be achieved, except for a small minority of the population, without a well-functioning health financing system. It determines whether people can afford to use health services when they need them. It determines if the services exist.

Recognizing this, Member States of the World Health Organization (WHO) committed in 2005 to develop their health financing systems so that all people have access to services and do not suffer financial hardship paying for them (4). This goal was defined as universal coverage, sometimes called universal health coverage.

In striving for this goal, governments face three fundamental questions:

1. How is such a health system to be financed?
2. How can they protect people from the financial consequences of ill-health and paying for health services?
3. How can they encourage the optimum use of available resources?

They must also ensure coverage is equitable and establish reliable means to monitor and evaluate progress.

In this report, WHO outlines how countries can modify their financing systems to move more quickly towards universal coverage and to sustain those achievements. The report synthesizes new research and lessons learnt from experience into a set of possible actions that countries at all stages of development can consider and adapt to their own needs. It suggests ways the international community can support efforts in low-income countries to achieve universal coverage.

As the world grapples with economic slowdown, globalization of diseases as well as economies, and growing demands for chronic care that are linked partly to ageing populations, the need for universal health coverage, and a strategy for financing it, has never been greater.

Where are we now?

The World Health Assembly resolution 58.33 from 2005 says everyone should be able to access health services and not be subject to financial hardship in doing so. On both counts, the world is still a long way from universal coverage.

On the service coverage side, the proportion of births attended by a skilled health worker can be as low as 10% in some countries, for example, while it is close to 100% for countries with the lowest rates of maternal mortality. Within countries, similar variations exist. Rich women generally obtain similar levels of coverage, wherever they live, but the poor miss out. Women in the richest 20% of the population are up to 20 times more likely to have a birth attended by a skilled health worker than a poor woman.

Closing this coverage gap between rich and poor in 49 low-income countries would save the lives of more than 700 000 women between now and 2015 (5). In the same vein, rich children live longer than poor ones; closing the coverage gap for a range of services for children under the age of five, particularly routine immunization, would save more than 16 million lives.

But income is not the only factor influencing service coverage. In many settings, migrants, ethnic minorities and indigenous people use services less than other population groups, even though their needs may be greater.

The other side of the coin is that when people do use services, they often incur high, sometimes catastrophic costs in paying for their care.

In some countries, up to 11% of the population suffers this type of severe financial hardship each year, and up to 5% is forced into poverty. Globally, about 150 million people suffer financial catastrophe annually while 100 million are pushed below the poverty line.

The other financial penalty imposed on the ill (and often their carers) is lost income. In most countries, relatives can provide some form of financial support, however small, to family members during periods of illness. More formal financial transfers to protect those too ill to work are less common. Only one in five people in the world has broad-based social security protection that also includes cover for lost wages in the event of illness, and more than half the world's population lacks any type of formal social protection, according to the International Labour Organization (ILO). Only 5–10% of people are covered in sub-Saharan Africa and southern Asia, while in middle-income countries, coverage rates range from 20% to 60%.

Health financing is an important part of broader efforts to ensure social protection in health. As such, WHO is joint lead agency with the ILO in the United Nations initiative to help countries develop a comprehensive Social Protection Floor, which includes the type of financial risk protection discussed in this report and the broader aspects of income replacement and social support in the event of illness (6).

How do we fix this?

Three fundamental, interrelated problems restrict countries from moving closer to universal coverage. The first is the availability of resources. No country, no matter how rich, has been able to ensure that everyone has immediate access to every technology and intervention that may improve their health or prolong their lives.

At the other end of the scale, in the poorest countries, few services are available to all.

The second barrier to universal coverage is an overreliance on direct payments at the time people need care. These include over-the-counter payments for medicines and fees for consultations and procedures. Even if people have some form of health insurance, they may need to contribute in the form of co-payments, co-insurance or deductibles.

The obligation to pay directly for services at the moment of need – whether that payment is made on a formal or informal (under the table) basis – prevents millions of people receiving health care when they need it. For those who do seek treatment, it can result in severe financial hardship, even impoverishment.

The third impediment to a more rapid movement towards universal coverage is the inefficient and inequitable use of resources. At a conservative estimate, 20–40% of health resources are being wasted. Reducing this waste would greatly improve the ability of health systems to provide quality services and improve health. Improved efficiency often makes it easier for the ministry of health to make a case for obtaining additional funding from the ministry of finance.

The path to universal coverage, then, is relatively simple – at least on paper. Countries must raise sufficient funds, reduce the reliance on direct payments to finance services, and improve efficiency and equity. These aspects are discussed in the next sections.

Many low- and middle-income countries have shown over the past decade that moving closer to universal coverage is not the prerogative of high-income countries. For example, Brazil, Chile, China, Mexico, Rwanda and Thailand have recently made great strides in addressing all three problems described above. Gabon has introduced innovative ways to raise funds for health, including a levy on mobile phone use; Cambodia has introduced a health equity fund that covers the health costs of the poor and Lebanon has improved the efficiency and quality of its primary care network.

Meanwhile, it is clear that every country can do more in at least one of the three key areas. Even high-income countries now realize they must continually reassess how they move forward in the face of rising costs and expectations. Germany, for example, has recognized its ageing population means wage and salary earners have declined as a proportion of the total population, making it more difficult to fund its social health insurance system from the traditional sources of wage-based insurance contributions. As a result, the government has injected additional funds from general revenues into the system.

Raising sufficient resources for health

Although domestic financial support for universal coverage will be crucial to its sustainability, it is unrealistic to expect most low-income countries to achieve universal coverage without help in the short term. The international community will need to financially support domestic efforts in the poorest countries to rapidly expand access to services.

For this to happen, it is important to know the likely cost. Recent estimates of the money needed to reach the health Millennium Development Goals (MDGs) and to ensure access to critical interventions, including for noncommunicable diseases in 49 low-income countries, suggest that, on average (unweighted), these countries will need to spend a little more than US$ 60 per capita by 2015, considerably more than the US$ 32 they are currently spending. This 2015 figure includes the cost of expanding the health system so that they can deliver the specified mix of interventions.

The first step to universal coverage, therefore, is to ensure that the poorest countries have these funds and that funding increases consistently over the coming years to enable the necessary scale-up.

But even countries currently spending more than the estimated minimum required cannot relax. Achieving the health MDGs and ensuring access to critical interventions focusing on noncommunicable diseases – the interventions included in the cost estimates reported here – is just the beginning. As the system improves, demands for more services, greater quality and/or higher levels of financial risk protection will inevitably follow. High-income countries are continually seeking funds to satisfy growing demands and expectations from their populations and to pay for rapidly expanding technologies and options for improving health.

All countries have scope to raise more money for health domestically, provided governments and the people commit to doing so. There are three broad ways to do this, plus a fourth option for increasing development aid and making it work better for health.

1. **Increase the efficiency of revenue collection**. Even in some high-income countries, tax avoidance and inefficient tax and insurance premium collection can be serious problems. The practical difficulties in collecting tax and health insurance contributions, particularly in countries with a large informal sector, are well documented. Improving the efficiency of revenue collection will increase the funds that can be used to provide services or buy them on behalf of the population. Indonesia has totally revamped its tax system with substantial benefits for overall government spending, and spending on health in particular.

2. **Reprioritize government budgets**. Governments sometimes give health a relatively low priority when allocating their budgets. For example, few African countries reach the target, agreed to by their heads of state in the 2001 Abuja Declaration, to spend 15% of their government budget on health; 19 of the countries in the region who signed the declaration allocate less now than they did in 2001. The United Republic of Tanzania, however, allots 18.4% to health and Liberia 16.6% (figures that include the contributions of external partners channelled through government, which are difficult to isolate). Taken as a group, the 49 low-income coun-

tries could raise an additional US$ 15 billion per year for health from domestic sources by increasing health's share of total government spending to 15%.

3. **Innovative financing**. Attention has until now focused largely on helping rich countries raise more funds for health in poor settings. The high-level Taskforce on Innovative International Financing for Health Systems included increasing taxes on air tickets, foreign exchange transactions and tobacco in its list of ways to raise an additional US$ 10 billion annually for global health. High-, middle- and low-income countries should all consider some of these mechanisms for domestic fundraising. A levy on foreign exchange transactions could raise substantial sums in some countries. India, for example, has a significant foreign exchange market, with daily turnover of US$ 34 billion. A currency transaction levy of 0.005% on this volume of trade could yield about US$ 370 million per year if India felt this path was appropriate. Other options include diaspora bonds (sold to expatriates) and solidarity levies on a range of products and services, such as mobile phone calls. Every tax has some type of distortionary effect on an economy and will be opposed by those with vested interests. Governments will need to implement those that best suit their economies and are likely to have political support. On the other hand, taxes on products that are harmful to health have the dual benefit of improving the health of the population through reduced consumption while raising more funds. A 50% increase in tobacco excise taxes would generate US$ 1.42 billion in additional funds in 22 low-income countries for which data are available. If all of this were allocated to health, it would allow government health spending to increase by more than 25% in several countries, and at the extreme, by 50%. Raising taxes on alcohol to 40% of the retail price could have an even bigger impact. Estimates for 12 low-income countries where data are available show that consumption levels would fall by more than 10%, while tax revenues would more than triple to a level amounting to 38% of total health spending in those countries. The potential to increase taxation on tobacco and alcohol exists in many countries. Even if only a portion of the proceeds were allocated to health, access to services would be greatly enhanced. Some countries are also considering taxes on other harmful products, such as sugary drinks and foods high in salt or transfats (7, 8).

4. **Development assistance for health.** While all countries, rich or poor, could do more to increase health funding or diversify their funding sources, only eight of the 49 low-income countries described earlier have any chance of generating from domestic sources alone the funds required to achieve the MDGs by 2015. Global solidarity is required. The funding shortfall faced by these low-income countries highlights the need for high-income countries to honour their commitments on official development assistance (ODA), and to back it up with greater effort to improve aid effectiveness. While innovative funding can supplement traditional ODA, if countries were to immediately keep their current international pledges, external funding for health in low-income countries would more than double overnight and the estimated shortfall in funds to reach the MDGs would be virtually eliminated.

Removing financial risks and barriers to access

While having sufficient funding is important, it will be impossible to get close to universal coverage if people suffer financial hardship or are deterred from using services because they have to pay on the spot. When this happens, the sick bear all of the financial risks associated with paying for care. They must decide if they can afford to receive care, and often this means choosing between paying for health services and paying for other essentials, such as food or children's education.

Where fees are charged, everyone pays the same price regardless of their economic status. There is no formal expression of solidarity between the sick and the healthy, or between the rich and the poor. Such systems make it impossible to spread costs over the life-cycle: paying contributions when one is young and healthy and drawing on them in the event of illness later in life. Consequently, the risk of financial catastrophe and impoverishment is high, and achieving universal coverage impossible.

Almost all countries impose some form of direct payment, sometimes called cost sharing, although the poorer the country, the higher the proportion of total expenditure that is financed in this way. The most extreme examples are found in 33 mostly low-income countries, where direct out-of-pocket payments represented more than 50% of total health expenditures in 2007.

The only way to reduce reliance on direct payments is for governments to encourage the risk-pooling, prepayment approach, the path chosen by most of the countries that have come closest to universal coverage. When a population has access to prepayment and pooling mechanisms, the goal of universal health coverage becomes more realistic. These are based on payments made in advance of an illness, pooled in some way and used to fund health services for everyone who is covered – treatment and rehabilitation for the sick and disabled, and prevention and promotion for everyone.

It is only when direct payments fall to 15–20% of total health expenditures that the incidence of financial catastrophe and impoverishment falls to negligible levels. It is a tough target, one that richer countries can aspire to, but other countries may wish to set more modest short-term goals. For example, the countries in the WHO South-East Asia and Western Pacific Regions recently set themselves a target of between 30% and 40%.

The funds can come from a variety of sources – income and wage-based taxes, broader-based value-added taxes or excise taxes on tobacco and alcohol, and/or insurance premiums. The source matters less than the policies developed to administer prepayment systems. Should these contributions be compulsory? Who should pay, how much and when? What should happen to people who cannot afford to contribute financially? Decisions also need to be taken on pooling. Should funds be kept as part of consolidated government revenues, or in one or more health insurance funds, be they social, private, community or micro funds?

Country experience reveals three broad lessons to be considered when formulating such policies.

First, in every country a proportion of the population is too poor to contribute via income taxes or insurance premiums. They will need to be subsidized from pooled funds, generally government revenues. Such assistance can take the form of direct access to government-financed services or through subsidies on their insurance premiums. Those countries whose entire populations have access to a set of services usually have relatively high levels of pooled funds – in the order of 5–6% of gross domestic product (GDP).

Second, contributions need to be compulsory, otherwise the rich and healthy will opt out and there will be insufficient funding to cover the needs of the poor and sick. While voluntary insurance schemes can raise some funds in the absence of widespread prepayment and pooling, and also help to familiarize people with the benefits of insurance, they have a limited ability to cover a range of services for those too poor to pay premiums. Longer-term plans for expanding prepayment and incorporating community and micro-insurance into the broader pool are important.

Third, pools that protect the health needs of a small number of people are not viable in the long run. A few episodes of expensive illness will wipe them out. Multiple pools, each with their own administrations and information systems, are also inefficient and make it difficult to achieve equity. Usually, one of the pools will provide high benefits to relatively wealthy people, who will not want to cross-subsidize the costs of poorer, less healthy people.

Cross-subsidization is possible where there are multiple funds, but this requires political will and technical and administrative capacities. In the Netherlands and Switzerland, for example, funds are transferred between insurance schemes that enrol people with few health needs (and who incur lower costs) to those enrolling high-risk people who require more services.

Even where funding is largely prepaid and pooled, there will need to be tradeoffs between the proportions of the population to be covered, the range of services to be made available and the proportion of the total costs to be met (Fig. 1). The box here labelled "current pooled funds" depicts the current situation in a hypothetical country, where about half the population is covered for about half of the possible services, but where less than half the cost of these services is met from pooled funds. To get closer to universal coverage, the country would need to extend coverage to more people, offer more services, and/or pay a greater part of the cost.

In countries with long-standing social health protection mechanisms such as those in Europe, or Japan, the current pooled funds box fills most of the space. But none of the high-income countries

Fig. 1. **Three dimensions to consider when moving towards universal coverage**

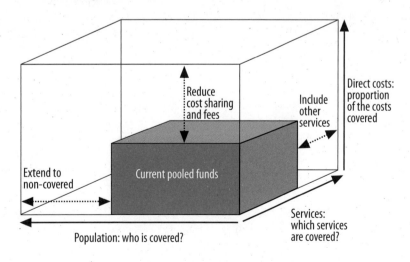

Source: Adapted from (9, 10).

that are commonly said to have achieved universal coverage actually covers 100% of the population for 100% of the services available and for 100% of the cost – and with no waiting lists. Each country fills the box in its own way, trading off the proportion of services and the proportion of the costs to be met from pooled funds.

Nevertheless, the entire population in all these countries has the right to use a set of services (prevention, promotion, treatment and rehabilitation). Virtually everyone is protected from severe financial risks thanks to funding mechanisms based on prepayment and pooling. The fundamentals are the same even if the specifics differ, shaped by the interplay of expectations between the population and the health providers, the political environment and the availability of funds.

Countries will take differing paths towards universal coverage, depending on where and how they start, and they will make different choices as they proceed along the three axes outlined in Fig. 1. For example, where all but the elite are excluded from health services, moving quickly towards a system that covers everyone, rich or poor, may be a priority, even if the list of services and the proportion of costs covered by pooled funds is relatively small. Meanwhile, in a broad-based system, with just a few pockets of exclusion, the country may initially take a targeted approach, identifying those that are excluded and taking steps to ensure they are covered. In such cases, they can cover more services to the poor and/or cover a higher proportion of the costs.

Ultimately, universal coverage requires a commitment to covering 100% of the population, and plans to this end need to be developed from the outset even if the objective will not be achieved immediately.

Other barriers to accessing health services

Removing the financial barriers implicit in direct-payment systems will help poorer people obtain care, but it will not guarantee it. Recent studies on why people do not complete treatment for chronic diseases show that transport costs and lost income can be even more prohibitive than the charges imposed for the service. Moreover, if services are not available at all or not available close by, people cannot use them even if they are free of charge.

Many countries are exploring ways to overcome these barriers. Conditional cash transfers, where people receive money if they do certain things to improve their health (usually linked to prevention), have increased the use of services in some cases. Other options include vouchers and refunds to cover transport costs, and microcredit schemes that allow members of poor households (often the women) the chance to earn money, which can be used in a variety of ways, including seeking or obtaining health services.

Promoting efficiency and eliminating waste

Raising sufficient money for health is imperative, but just having the money will not ensure universal coverage. Nor will removing financial barriers to access through prepayment and pooling. The final requirement is to ensure resources are used efficiently.

Opportunities to achieve more with the same resources exist in all countries. Expensive medicines are often used when cheaper, equally effective options are available. In many settings, antibiotics and injections are overused, there is poor storage and wastage, and wide variations in the prices procurement agencies negotiate with suppliers. Reducing unnecessary expenditure on medicines and using them more appropriately, and improving quality control, could save countries up to 5% of their health expenditure.

Medicines account for three of the most common causes of inefficiency outlined in this report. Solutions for the other six can be grouped under the following headings:

- Get the most out of technologies and health services
- Motivate health workers
- Improve hospital efficiency
- Get care right the first time by reducing medical errors
- Eliminate waste and corruption
- Critically assess what services are needed.

Conservatively speaking, about 20–40% of resources spent on health are wasted, resources that could be redirected towards achieving universal coverage.

All countries, no matter what their income level, can take steps to reduce inefficiency, something that requires an initial assessment of the nature and causes of local inefficiencies drawing on the analysis in this report. Inefficiency can sometimes be due to insufficient, rather than too much, spending on health. For example, low salaries result in health workers supplementing their income by working a second job concurrently, reducing output for their primary employment. It is then necessary to assess the costs and likely impact of the possible solutions.

Incentives for greater efficiency can be built into the way service providers are paid. Fee-for-service payment encourages over-servicing for those who can afford to pay or whose costs are met from pooled funds (e.g. taxes and insurance), and underservicing for those who cannot pay.

Many alternatives have been tried. All have advantages and disadvantages. Where fee-for-service is the norm, governments and insurance companies have had to introduce controls to reduce over-servicing. These controls can be costly to implement, requiring additional human capacity and infrastructure to measure and monitor the use (and possible overuse) of services.

In other settings, fee-for-service payments have been replaced by capitation at the primary-care level, or by some form of case-based payment, such as diagnostic-related groups at the hospital level. Capitation involves payment of a fixed sum per person enrolled with a provider or facility in each time period, regardless of the services provided. Case-base payment is for a fixed sum per case, again regardless of the intensity or duration of hospital treatment.

Both reduce incentives for over-servicing. However, it has been argued diagnostic-related groups (i.e. payment of a standard rate for a procedure, regardless of how long patients stay in hospital) may encourage hospitals to discharge patients early, then to re-admit rapidly, thereby incurring two payments instead of one.

Paying service providers is a complex, ever-changing process and some countries have developed a mixed payment system, believing it is more efficient than a single payment mode.

It is possible to find more efficient approaches to purchasing services, often described as strategic purchasing. The traditional system in which providers are reimbursed for their services (and national governments allocate budgets to various levels of administration based largely on the funding they received the previous year) has been termed passive purchasing. More active purchasing can improve quality and efficiency by asking explicit questions about the population's health needs: what interventions and services best meet these needs and expectations given the available resources? What is the appropriate mix of promotion, prevention, treatment and rehabilitation? How and from whom should these interventions and services be purchased and provided?

Strategic purchasing is more than making a simple choice between passive and active purchasing. Countries will decide where they can operate based on their ability to collect, monitor and interpret the necessary information, and to encourage and enforce standards of quality and efficiency. Passive purchasing creates inefficiency. The closer countries can move towards active purchasing, the more efficient the system is likely to be.

Inequalities in coverage

Governments have a responsibility to ensure that all providers, public and private, operate appropriately and attend to patients' needs cost effectively and efficiently. They also must ensure that a range of population-based services focusing on prevention and promotion is available, services such as mass communication programmes designed to reduce tobacco consumption, or to encourage mothers to take their children to be immunized.

They are also responsible for ensuring that everyone can obtain the services they need and that all are protected from the financial risks associated with using them. This can conflict with the drive towards efficiency, for the most efficient way of using resources is not always the most equitable. For example, it is usually more efficient to locate services in populated areas, but reaching the rural poor will require locating services closer to them.

Governments must also be aware that free public services may be captured by the rich, who use them more than the poor, even though their need may be less. In some countries, only the richest people have access to an adequate level of services, while in others, only the poorest are excluded. Some groups of people slip through the gaps in most systems, and patterns of exclusion from services vary. Particular attention must be paid to the difficulties women and ethnic and migrant groups face in accessing services, and to the special problems experienced by indigenous populations.

An agenda for action

No country starts from scratch in the way it finances health care. All have some form of system in place, and must build on it according to their values, constraints and opportunities. This process should be informed by national and international experience.

All countries can do more to raise funds for health or to diversify their sources of funding, to reduce the reliance on direct payments by promoting prepayment and pooling, and to use funds more efficiently and equitably, provided the political will exists.

Health can be a trailblazer in increasing efficiency and equity. Decision-makers in health can do a great deal to reduce leakage, for example, notably in procurement. They can also take steps, including regulation and legislation, to improve service delivery and the overall efficiency of the system – steps that other sectors could then follow.

Simply choosing from a menu of options, or importing what has worked in other settings, will not be sufficient. Health financing strategy needs to be home-grown, pushing towards universal coverage out of existing terrain. It is imperative, therefore, that countries develop their capacities to analyse and understand the strengths and weaknesses of the system in place so that they can adapt health financing policies accordingly, implement them, and monitor and modify them over time.

Facilitating and supporting change

The lessons described above focus on the technical challenges of health financing reform. But the technical aspect is only one component of policy development and implementation; a variety of accompanying actions that facilitate reflection and change are necessary.

These actions are captured in the health financing decision process represented in Fig. 2. It is intended as a guide rather than a blueprint, and it should be noted that while the processes we envisage are represented as conceptually discrete, they overlap and evolve on an ongoing basis.

The seven actions described here apply not only to low- and middle-income countries. High-income countries that have achieved elevated levels of financial risk protection and coverage also need to continuously self-assess to ensure the financing system achieves its objectives in the face of ever-changing diagnostic and treatment practices and technologies, increasing demands and fiscal constraints.

Devising and implementing health finance strategy is a process of continuous adaptation, rather than linear progress towards some notional perfection. It must start with a clear statement of the principles and ideals driving the financing system – an understanding of what universal health coverage means in the particular country. This prepares the ground for the situation analysis (action 2). Action 3 identifies the financial envelope and how this is likely to change over time. It includes consideration of how much people are paying out of pocket and how much is spent in the nongovernmental sector. Action 4 considers the potential constraints on

developing and implementing plans to move closer to universal coverage, while actions 5 and 6 cover the formulation and implementation of detailed strategies.

The cycle, as we envisage it, is completed (action 7) when a country reviews its progress towards its stated goals (action 1), allowing its strategies to be re-evaluated and new plans made to redress any problems. It is a process based on continual learning, the practical realities of the system feeding constant re-evaluation and adjustment.

Health financing systems must adapt, and not just because there is always room for improvement, but because the countries they serve also change: disease patterns evolve, resources ebb and flow, institutions develop or decline.

Fig. 2. **The health financing decision process**

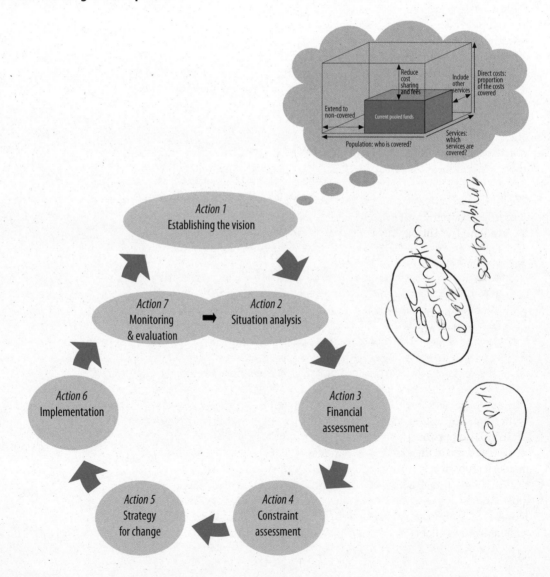

Practical steps for external partners

As noted above, many of the poorest countries will be unable for many years to finance a system of universal coverage – even one with a modest set of health services – from their own domestic resources. To allow the poorest countries to scale up more rapidly, external partners will need to increase contributions to meet their previously agreed international commitments. This act alone would close almost all the financing gap identified for 49 low-income countries earlier, and save more than 3 million additional lives before 2015.

Traditional ODA can be supplemented by innovative sources of funding. As the high-level taskforce suggested, some of the innovative ways to raise funds discussed earlier could also be applied at the international level. Some are already being implemented, as evidenced by the Millennium Foundation's MassiveGood campaign. Many innovative financing mechanisms do not require international consensus. If each high-income country introduced just one of the options that have been discussed, it could raise serious levels of additional funding to support a more rapid movement towards universal coverage in the countries most in need.

External partners could also help to strengthen the financing systems in recipient countries. Donors currently use multiple funding channels that add considerably to the transaction costs at both the country and international level. Harmonizing systems would put an end to the many auditing, monitoring and evaluation mechanisms competing with domestic systems for accountants, auditors, and actuaries. It would also free health ministry and other government staff to spend more time extending health coverage.

The international community has made progress by adopting the Paris Declaration on Aid Effectiveness and the subsequent Accra Agenda for Action. The International Health Partnership and related initiatives seek to implement the principles laid out in the declaration and the agenda. However, much remains to be done. Viet Nam reports that in 2009 there were more than 400 donor missions to review health projects or the health sector. Rwanda has to report annually on 890 health indicators to various donors, 595 relating to HIV and malaria alone while new global initiatives with secretariats are being created.

A message of hope

The first key message of this world health report is that there is no magic bullet to achieving universal access. Nevertheless, a wide range of experiences from around the world suggests that countries can move forward faster than they have done in the past or take actions to protect the gains that have been made. It is possible to raise additional funds and to diversify funding sources. It is possible to move away from direct payments towards prepayment and pooling (or to ensure that efforts to contain the growth of expenditures do not, in fact, extend the reliance on direct payments) and to become more efficient and equitable in the use of resources.

The principles are well established. Lessons have been learned from the countries that have put these principles into practice. Now is the time to take those lessons and build on them, for there is scope for every country to do something to speed up or sustain progress towards universal coverage. ■

References

1. *A global look at public perceptions of health problems, priorities, and donors: the Kaiser/Pew global health survey.* The Henry J Kaiser Family Foundation, 2007 (http://www.kff.org/kaiserpolls/upload/7716.pdf, accessed 23 June 2010).

2. Eurobaromètre standard 72: l'opinion publique dans l'Union Européenne, 2010 (http://ec.europa.eu/public_opinion/archives/eb/eb72/eb72_vol1_fr.pdf, accessed 23 June 2010).

3. *Closing the gap in a generation – health equity through action on the social determinants of health.* Geneva, World Health Organization, 2008 (http://whqlibdoc.who.int/hq/2008/WHO_IER_CSDH_08.1_eng.pdf, accessed 23 June 2010).

4. Resolution WHA58.33. Sustainable health financing, universal coverage and social health insurance. In: *Fifty-eighth World Health Assembly, Geneva, 16–25 May 2005.* Geneva, World Health Organization, 2005 (http://apps.who.int/gb/ebwha/pdf_files/WHA58/WHA58_33-en.pdf, accessed 23 June 2010).

5. Taskforce on Innovative International Financing for Health Systems, Working Group 1. WHO background paper: constraints to scaling up and costs. International Health Partnership, 2009 (http://www.internationalhealthpartnership.net/pdf/IHP%20Update%2013/Taskforce/Johansbourg/Working%20Group%201%20Report%20%20Final.pdf, accessed 23 June 2010).

6. *World social security report 2010/11: providing coverage in the time of crisis and beyond.* Geneva, International Labour Organization, 2010.

7. Leonhardt D. The battle over taxing soda. *The New York Times*, 18 May 2010, B:1.

8. Holt E. Romania mulls over fast food tax. *Lancet*, 2010,375:1070- doi:10.1016/S0140-6736(10)60462-X PMID:20352658

9. *The world health report 2008: primary health care – now more than ever.* Geneva, World Health Organization, 2008.

10. Busse R, Schlette S, eds. *Focus on prevention, health and aging, new health professions.* Gütersloh, Verlag Bertelsmann Stiftung, 2007.

End notes

a   In this report, the term "health services" is used to include promotion, prevention, treatment and rehabilitation. It includes services aimed at individuals (e.g. childhood immunization or treatment for tuberculosis) and services aimed at populations (e.g. mass media anti-smoking campaigns).

Chapter 1 | Where are we now?

co-produce.

Key messages

- Improving health is critical to human welfare and essential to sustained economic and social development. Reaching the "highest attainable standard of health," as stated in the WHO Constitution, requires a new or continued drive towards universal coverage in many countries, and strong actions to protect the gains that have been achieved in others.

- To achieve universal health coverage, countries need financing systems that enable people to use all types of health services – promotion, prevention, treatment and rehabilitation – without incurring financial hardship.

- Today, millions of people cannot use health services because they have to pay for them at the time they receive them. And many of those who do use services suffer financial hardship, or are even impoverished, because they have to pay.

- Moving away from direct payments at the time services are received to prepayment is an important step to averting the financial hardship associated with paying for health services. Pooling the resulting funds increases access to needed services, and spreads the financial risks of ill health across the population.

- Pooled funds will never be able to cover 100% of the population for 100% of the costs and 100% of needed services. Countries will still have to make hard choices about how best to use these funds.

- Globally, we are a long way from achieving universal health coverage. But countries at all income levels have recently made important progress towards that goal by raising more funds for health, pooling them more effectively to spread financial risks, and becoming more efficient.

1

Where are we now?

The accident happened on 7 October 2006. Narin Pintalakarn came off his motorcycle going into a bend. He struck a tree, his unprotected head taking the full force of the impact. Passing motorists found him some time later and took him to a nearby hospital. Doctors diagnosed severe head injury and referred him to the trauma centre, 65 km away, where the diagnosis was confirmed. A scan showed subdural haematoma with subfalcine and uncal herniation. Pintalakarn's skull had fractured in several places. His brain had bulged and shifted, and was still bleeding; the doctors decided to operate. He was wheeled into an emergency department where a surgeon removed part of his skull to relieve pressure. A blood clot was also removed. Five hours later, the patient was put on a respirator and taken to the intensive care unit where he stayed for 21 days. Thirty-nine days after being admitted to hospital, he had recovered sufficiently to be discharged.

What is remarkable about this story is not what it says about the power of modern medicine to repair a broken body; it is remarkable because the episode took place not in a country belonging to the Organisation for Economic Co-operation and Development (OECD), where annual per capita expenditure on health averages close to US$ 4000, but in Thailand, a country that spends US$ 136 per capita, just 3.7% of its gross domestic product (GDP) (1). Nor did the patient belong to the ruling elite, the type of person who – as this report shall show – tends to get good treatment wherever they live. Pintalakarn was a casual labourer, earning only US$ 5 a day.

"Thai legislation demands that all injured patients be taken care of with standard procedure no matter what their status," says Dr Witaya Chadbunchachai, the surgeon who carried out the craniotomy on Pintalakarn at the Khon Kaen Regional Hospital in the country's north-eastern province. According to Chadbunchachai, medical staff do not consider who is going to pay for treatment, however expensive it might be, because in Thailand, everyone's health-care costs are covered.

At a time when many countries, including major economic powers such as China and the United States of America, are reviewing the way they meet the health-care needs of their populations, universal health coverage – what is it, how much does it cost and how is it to be paid for? – dominates discussions on health service provision. In this world health report, we examine the issue from the financing perspective, and suggest ways in which all countries, rich and poor, can improve access to good quality health services without people experiencing financial hardship because they must pay for care (Box 1.1).

The three critical areas of health financing are:

1. raise sufficient money for health;
2. remove financial barriers to access and reduce financial risks of illness;
3. make better use of the available resources (Box 1.1 provides details).

Box 1.1. **What a health financing system does: a technical explanation**

Health financing is much more than a matter of raising money for health. It is also a matter of who is asked to pay, when they pay, and how the money raised is spent.

Revenue collection is what most people associate with health financing: the way money is raised to pay health system costs. Money is typically received from households, organizations or companies, and sometimes from contributors outside the country (called "external sources"). Resources can be collected through general or specific taxation; compulsory or voluntary health insurance contributions; direct out-of-pocket payments, such as user fees; and donations.

Pooling is the accumulation and management of financial resources to ensure that the financial risk of having to pay for health care is borne by all members of the pool and not by the individuals who fall ill. The main purpose of pooling is to spread the financial risk associated with the need to use health services. If funds are to be pooled, they have to be *prepaid*, before the illness occurs – through taxes and/or insurance, for example. Most health financing systems include an element of pooling funded by prepayment, combined with direct payments from individuals to service providers, sometimes called *cost-sharing*.

Purchasing is the process of paying for health services. There are three main ways to do this. One is for government to provide budgets directly to its own health service providers (integration of purchasing and provision) using general government revenues and, sometimes, insurance contributions. The second is for an institutionally separate purchasing agency (e.g. a health insurance fund or government authority) to purchase services on behalf of a population (a purchaser-provider split). The third is for individuals to pay a provider directly for services. Many countries use a combination.

Within these broad areas, health service providers can be paid in many different ways, discussed more fully in Chapter 4. Purchasing also includes deciding which services should be financed, including the mix between prevention, promotion, treatment and rehabilitation. This is addressed further in Chapter 2.

Labels can be misleading. Each country makes different choices about how to raise revenues, how to pool them and how to purchase services. The fact that several countries decide to raise part of the revenue for health from compulsory health insurance premiums does not mean that they all pool the funds in the same way. Some countries have a single pool – e.g. a national health insurance fund – while others have multiple, sometimes competing pools managed by private insurance companies. Even when countries have similar pooling systems, their choices about how to provide or purchase services vary considerably. Two systems based largely on health insurance may operate differently in how they pool funds and use them to ensure that people can access services; the same applies to two systems that are described as tax-based. This is why the traditional categorization of financing systems into tax-based and social health insurance – or Beveridge versus Bismarck – is no longer useful for policy-making.

It is much more important to consider the choices to be made at each step along the path, from raising revenues, to pooling them, to spending them. These are the choices that determine whether a financing system is going to be effective, efficient and equitable, choices that are described in the subsequent chapters.

People at the centre. In all of this technical work, it is important to remember that people are at the centre. On the one hand, they provide the funds required to pay for services. On the other, the only reason for raising these funds is to improve people's health and welfare. Health financing is a means to an end, not an end in itself.

Health services cost money. One way or another, doctors and nurses, medicines and hospitals have to be paid for. Today, global annual expenditure on health is about US$ 5.3 trillion (*1*). With the burden of communicable diseases remaining stubbornly high in some parts of the world, and the prevalence of noncommunicable diseases – heart disease, cancers and chronic conditions such as obesity – increasing everywhere, health costs can only continue to rise. This trend will be exacerbated by the more sophisticated medicines and procedures being developed to treat them.

It would seem logical, therefore, that richer countries are better able to provide affordable health services. Indeed, the countries that have come closest to achieving universal coverage do generally have more to spend on health. OECD countries, for example, represent only 18% of the global population but account for 86% of the world's health spending; few OECD countries spend less than US$ 2900 per person each year.

But it is not always the case that lower-income countries have less coverage. Thailand is a striking example of a country that has vastly improved service coverage and protection against the financial risks of ill health despite spending much less on health than higher-income countries. It has done this by changing the way it raises funds for health and moving away from direct payments, such as user fees (Box 1.2). This is perhaps the most crucial element of developing financing systems for universal coverage; many countries still rely too heavily on direct payments from individuals to health service providers to fund their health systems.

Direct payments

Direct payments have serious repercussions for health. Making people pay at the point of delivery discourages them from using services (particularly health promotion and prevention), and encourages them to postpone health checks. This means they do not receive treatment early, when the prospects for cure are greatest. It has been estimated that a high proportion of the world's 1.3 billion poor have no access to health services simply because they cannot afford to pay at the time they need them (*2*). They risk being pushed into poverty, or further into poverty, because they are too ill to work.

Direct payments also hurt household finances. Many people who do seek treatment, and have to pay for it at the point of delivery, suffer severe financial difficulties as a consequence (*3–6*). Estimates of the number of people who suffer financial catastrophe (defined as paying more than 40% of household income directly on health care after basic needs have been met) are available for 89 countries, covering nearly 90% of the world's population (*7*). In some countries, up to 11% of people suffer this type of severe financial hardship each year and up to 5% are forced into poverty because they must pay for health services at the time they receive them. Recent studies show that these out-of-pocket health payments pushed 100 000 households in both Kenya and Senegal below the poverty line in a single year. About 290 000 experienced the same fate in South Africa (*8*).

Financial catastrophe occurs in countries at all income levels, but is greatest in those that rely the most on direct payments to raise funds for health (*9*). Worldwide, about 150 million people a year face catastrophic health-care costs because of direct payments such as user fees, while 100 million are driven below the poverty line (*7*).

Catastrophic health spending is not necessarily caused by high-cost medical procedures or one single expensive event. For many households, relatively small payments can also result in financial catastrophe (*10*). A steady drip of medical bills can force people with chronic disease or disabilities, for example, into poverty (*11–13*).

Not only do out-of-pocket payments deter people from using health services and cause financial stress, they also cause inefficiency and inequity in the way resources are used. They encourage overuse by people who can pay and underuse by those who cannot (Box 1.3).

Box 1.2. What are direct payments?

In health, charges or fees are commonly levied for consultations with health professionals, medical or investigative procedures, medicines and other supplies, and for laboratory tests.

Depending on the country, they are levied by government, nongovernmental organizations, faith-based and private health facilities.

They are sometimes officially sanctioned charges and sometimes unofficial or so-called "under-the-table" payments. Sometimes both co-exist.

Even where these charges are covered by insurance, patients are generally required to share the costs, typically in the form of co-insurance, co-payments and/or deductibles – payments the insured person has to make directly out of pocket at the time they use services because these costs are not covered by the insurance plan.

Deductibles are the amount of expenses that must be paid out of pocket before an insurer will cover any expenses at all. Co-insurance reflects the proportion of subsequent costs that must be met out of pocket by the person who is covered, while co-payments are set as a fixed amount the beneficiary must pay for each service.

We use the term *direct payments* to capture all these elements. However, because the term *out-of-pocket payments* is often used to capture the same ideas, we use the two terms interchangeably.

Pooled funds

Progress towards universal coverage depends on raising adequate funds from a sufficiently large pool of individuals, supplemented where necessary with donor support and general government revenues, and spending these funds on the services a population needs. The more people who share the financial risk in this way, the lower the financial risk to which any one individual is exposed. In general, the bigger the pool, the better able it is to cope with financial risks. Using the same reasoning, pools with only a few participants are likely to experience what actuaries term "extreme fluctuations in utilization and claims" (16).

For a pool to exist, money must be put into it, which is why a system of prepayment is required. Prepayment simply means that people pay before they are sick, then draw on the pooled funds when they fall ill. There are different ways of organizing prepayment for the people who can afford to pay (see Chapter 3) but in all countries there will be people who are unable to contribute financially. The countries that have come closest to achieving universal health coverage use tax revenue to cover the health needs to these people, ensuring that everyone can access services when they need them.

Countries are at different points on the path to universal coverage and at different stages of developing financing systems. Rwanda, for example, has a tax system that is still developing, and three robust health insurance organizations (Box 1.4). It may decide to build larger pools by merging the individual funds at a later date.

External assistance

In lower-income countries, where prepayment structures may be underdeveloped or inefficient and where health needs are massive, there are many obstacles to raising sufficient funds through prepayment and pooling. It is essential, therefore, that international donors lend their support. Investing in the development of prepayment and pooling, as opposed to simply funding projects or programmes through separate channels, is one of the best ways donors can help countries move away from user fees and improve access to health care and financial risk protection (21, 22).

Over the past five years, many bilateral agencies have begun to help countries develop their health financing systems, with a view to achieving universal coverage. These agencies have also started to determine how their external financial assistance can support, rather than hinder this process. This is reflected in the adoption of the Paris Declaration on Aid Effectiveness and the subsequent Accra Action Agenda. The International Health Partnership and related initiatives

Box 1.3. **Financing for universal health coverage**

Financing systems need to be specifically designed to:

- provide all people with access to needed health services (including prevention, promotion, treatment and rehabilitation) of sufficient quality to be effective;
- ensure that the use of these services does not expose the user to financial hardship (14).

In 2005, the World Health Assembly unanimously adopted a resolution urging countries to develop their health financing systems to achieve these two goals, defined then as achieving universal coverage (15). The more that countries rely on direct payments, such as user-fees, to fund their health systems, the more difficult is it to meet these two objectives.

seek to implement these principles into practice in the health sector, with the aim to mobilize donor countries and other development partners around a single, country-led national health strategy (*23, 24*).

On the path to universal coverage

Many countries are reforming the way they finance health care as they move towards universal coverage, among them two of the most important global economies, China and the United States of America.

In April 2009, the Chinese government announced plans to provide "safe, effective, convenient and affordable" health services to all urban and rural residents by 2020 (*25*). If fully implemented, the reform will end market-based mechanisms for health that were introduced in 1978. Prior to then, the government had offered basic but essentially free health-care services to the entire population, but the new market-based approach resulted in a major increase in direct payments – from little more than 20% of all health spending in 1980 to 60% in 2000 – leaving many people facing catastrophic health-care costs. The new approach also meant that hospitals had to survive on patient fees, which put pressure on doctors to prescribe medicines and treatment based on their revenue-generating potential rather than their clinical efficacy.

The government took steps to address these issues. The New Cooperative Medical Schemes, initiated in 2003 to meet the needs of rural populations, and the Urban Residents Basic Medical Insurance scheme, piloted in 79 cities in 2007, are at the heart of the latest reforms. The government aims to reduce dependence on direct payments and increase the proportion of the population covered by formal insurance from 15% in 2003 to 90% by 2011, and to expand access to services and financial risk protection over time (*26*).

The recent health financing reforms in the United States will extend insurance coverage to a projected 32 million previously uninsured people by 2019 (*27*). Numerous strategies will be used to achieve this goal. Private insurers will no longer be able to reject applicants based on health status, for example, and low-income individuals and families will have their premiums subsidized (*28*).

Many low- to middle-income countries have also made significant progress developing their financing systems towards universal coverage.

Box 1.4. Sharing the risk of sickness: mutual health insurance in Rwanda

The Rwandan government reports that 91% of the country's population belongs to one of three principal health insurance schemes (*17*). The first, the *Rwandaise assurance maladie*, is a compulsory social health insurance scheme for government employees that is also open to private-sector employees on a voluntary basis. The second, the Military Medical Insurance scheme, covers the needs of all military personnel. The third, and most important for population coverage, is the cluster of *Assurances maladies communautaires* – mutual insurance schemes whose members predominantly live in rural settings and work in the informal sector. These mutual insurance schemes have expanded rapidly over the past 10 years, and now cover more than 80% of the population. About 50% of mutual insurance scheme funding comes from member premiums, the other half being subsidized by the government through a mix of general tax revenues and donor support (*18*).

The insurance schemes do not cover all health costs: households still have to pay a proportion of their costs out of pocket and the range of services available is clearly not as extensive as in richer countries. Nevertheless, they have had a marked impact. Per capita spending on health went up from US$ 11 in 1999 to US$ 37 in 2007; the increasing proportion of the population covered by some form of health insurance has translated into increased uptake of health services, and, most important of all, to improvements in health outcomes measured, for example, by declines in child mortality (*19*).

At an early stage of its development, challenges still exist. These include: making contributions more affordable for the poorest; increasing the range of services offered and the proportion of total costs covered; and improving financial management. Rwanda is also working to harmonize the different financing mechanisms, partly through the development of a national legal framework governing social health insurance (*20*).

These include well-known examples, such as Chile (*29*), Colombia (*6*), Cuba (*30*), Rwanda (*20*), Sri Lanka (*31*) and Thailand (*32*), but also Brazil (*33*), Costa Rica (*34*), Ghana (*35*), Kyrgyzstan (*36*), Mongolia (*37*) and the Republic of Moldova (*38*). At the same time, Gabon (*39*), the Lao People's Democratic Republic (*40*), Mali (*41*), the Philippines (*42*), Tunisia (*43*) and Viet Nam (*44*) have expanded various forms of prepayment and pooling to increase financial risk protection, particularly for the poor.

At the other end of the income scale, 27 OECD countries cover all their citizens with a set of interventions from pooled funds, while two others – Mexico, with its *Seguro Popular* voluntary health insurance scheme, and Turkey, with its Health Transformation Programme – are moving towards it (*45–47*).

Each of these countries has moved towards universal coverage in different ways and at different speeds. Sometimes their systems have evolved over long periods, often in the face of opposition; sometimes the path has been shorter and quicker (*21, 48*).

The Republic of Korea, for example, started its journey in the early 1960s. Early investment focused on building infrastructure, but the programme expanded significantly in 1977 with vigorous high-level political support (*49*). Steady expansion of employer-based health-care schemes followed, starting with companies employing more than 500 staff, moving down the corporate chain to companies employing just 16, and more recently to those with only one full-time employee. Civil servants and teachers were brought into the scheme in 1981 and played a key role in raising awareness in the rest of the population. This, in turn, helped put universal coverage at the heart of the political agenda in 1988, when enrolment in social welfare programmes was a core issue in the presidential campaign. In 1989, coverage was extended to the remaining population – the indigent, the self-employed and rural residents (*50*). Since then, the system has sought to expand both the range of services offered and the proportion of the costs covered by the insurance system.

Sustaining existing achievements

Moving more rapidly towards universal coverage is one challenge, but sustaining gains already made can be equally difficult. Several countries have adapted their financing systems in the face of changing circumstances. Ghana, for example, began after independence in 1957 to provide medical care to its population free at the point of service through government-funded facilities. It abandoned this system in the early 1980s in the face of severe resource constraints, before introducing a form of national insurance more recently (Box 1.5).

Chile, too, has gone through different phases. After running a state-funded national health service for 30 years, it opted in 2000 for a mixed public/private approach to health insurance, guaranteeing universal access to quality treatment for a set of explicitly defined conditions. The number of conditions has expanded over time and the poor have been the major beneficiaries (*29*).

All countries face increasing demands for better services, disease threats and a growing list of often expensive technologies and medicines to maintain or improve health. Costs continually rise faster than national income, putting pressure on governments to restrain costs.

Universal coverage: the two prongs

Many countries, at varying stages of economic development, have shown it is possible to make substantial progress towards universal coverage. Nevertheless, the world as a whole still has a long way to go. To learn where we stand today, we must focus on the two key elements of universal health coverage described earlier: financial access to crucial health services; and the extent of financial risk protection provided to the people who use them (Box 1.3).

As mentioned earlier, an estimated 150 million people globally suffer financial catastrophe each year and 100 million are pushed into poverty because of direct payments for health services. This indicates a widespread lack of financial risk protection – a deficiency that affects low-income countries most, but is by no means limited to them. In six of the OECD countries, more than 1% of the population, or almost four million people, suffers catastrophic spending, while the incidence exceeds five per 1000 people in another five (7).

Furthermore, medical debt is the principal cause of personal bankruptcy in the USA. Harvard researchers in 2008 concluded that illness or medical bills had contributed to 62% of bankruptcies the previous year (52). Many of these people had some form of health insurance, but the benefits offered were insufficient to protect them against high out-of-pocket expenses. This development is not linked to the recent economic recession; medical bills were already the cause of 50% of bankruptcies in the USA in 2001.

On a global scale, medical bankruptcies are not yet a major concern, either because financial access to care is adequate or because formal credit is out of the reach of most of the population (53, 54). However, if direct payments remain high and access to credit increases, this is likely to become a problem.

The reduction in the incidence of financial hardship associated with direct payments is a key indicator of progress towards universal coverage. However, country studies sometimes indicate little financial catastrophe or impoverishment of this nature among the most poor, because they simply cannot afford to use health services (55, 56). The extent to which people are able to use needed services is, therefore, also an important indicator of the health of the financing system.

Box 1.5. Ghana: different phases of health financing reforms

After independence in 1957, Ghana provided medical care to its population through a network of primary-care facilities. The system was financed through general taxation and received a degree of external donor support. No fees were charged for services. In the 1980s, faced with worsening economic conditions, the country liberalized its health sector as part of broader structural reforms. Liberalization led to an explosion in the number of private health-care providers, which, combined with the introduction of fees to cover part of the costs of government facilities, led to a sharp drop in the use of health services, particularly among the poor. Those people who did seek treatment paid out of their own pocket often risked financial ruin as a result (51).

More recently, out-of-pocket payment has started to decrease as a proportion of total health expenditure as the country tries to reverse these developments. The process began with exemptions from user fees for diseases such as leprosy and tuberculosis, and for immunization and antenatal care. Ghana also waives fees for people with extremely low incomes. A National Health Insurance Scheme was introduced in 2004 and by June 2009, 67.5% of the population had registered (35). During the 2005–2008 period, national outpatient-care visits increased by 50%, from about 12 million to 18 million, while inpatient-care admissions increased by 6.3%, from 0.8 million to about 0.85 million.

For the time being, each of the district mutual health insurance schemes that comprise the national scheme effectively constitutes a separate risk pool. Fragmentation is thus a continuing problem, as is sustainability, but Ghana is committed to redressing the move away from universal coverage over the past few decades.

Data on financial access to health services are scarce, but there is information on coverage for some key interventions. This provides clues on the extent to which financial barriers prevent people from using services. For example, immunizing children under one year of age with the diphtheria–tetanus–pertussis vaccine (DTP3) saves many of their lives, while having skilled health personnel attend births is crucial to saving the lives of both new-borns and mothers. Information on the proportion of children fully immunized with DTP3 and the proportion of births attended by skilled health personnel is widely reported.

Fig. 1.1 shows reported coverage for both of these interventions, with each data point representing a country, ordered from lowest to highest on the horizontal axis. Many countries achieve, or almost achieve, 100% coverage for both interventions, though there is considerable variation across countries. At one extreme, in 16 countries, fewer than 40% of women deliver babies in the presence of a skilled health worker capable of saving their lives in the event of a complication. In seven countries, DTP3 immunization coverage is lower than 40%. This suggests that inequalities in coverage are substantial across countries and greater for services that require more infrastructure and skilled workers (such as childbirth) than for other interventions (such as vaccinations) (57).

Inequalities in coverage (and health outcomes) also exist within countries. Demographic and Health Surveys reveal substantial differences between income groups in many lower-income countries. Again, bigger discrepancies occur in access to skilled health workers during child delivery than in childhood immunization. With few exceptions, the richest people in even low-income countries enjoy access to services similar to that available in high-income countries. The poor, however, are almost always more deprived than the rich, though the extent varies. In some settings, coverage of DTP3 among the poor can be as low as 10% of that for the rich (58).

The use of health services also varies substantially across and within countries (59, 60). Data from the 52 countries included in the World Health Survey, spanning all income levels, showed that usage during a four-week period before the survey ranged from less than 10% of the population to more than 30% (58). In some settings, the rich reported using these services more than twice as much as the poor, despite the fact the poor need them much more.

While the data cited give an indication of coverage, they offer no insight into the quality of care. What

Fig. 1.1. **Coverage of births attended by skilled health personnel and diphtheria–tetanus–pertussis (DTP3) vaccination by country, latest available year[a]**

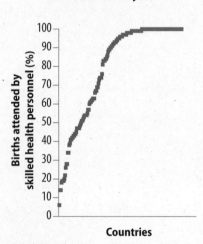

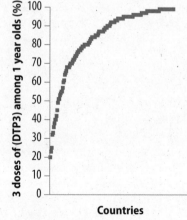

[a] Ordered from lowest to highest coverage.
Source: (19).

evidence does exist suggests that the inequalities are even more pronounced in the standard of service provided. In other words, poor people in poor countries are not only largely excluded from these services, but when they do receive care, it is likely to be of a lower quality than that provided to richer people (61).

These broad indications offer a sobering picture, one in which millions of people, predominantly poor, cannot use the services they need, while millions more face severe financial difficulty as a result of paying for health services. Clearly, the reasons for low and unequal coverage do not all lie in the financing system, but we argue in this report that coverage could be considerably higher if there were additional funds, less reliance on direct payments to raise funds and more efficiency – all financing issues.

Several countries increase financial risk protection beyond that afforded by the health financing system by providing an element of financial security when people cannot work for health reasons – because they are sick or have had a baby. The International Labour Organization (ILO) collates information on the right to paid sick leave in the event of illness as well as on the right to paid maternity leave. In 2007, 145 countries provided the right to paid sick leave, although the duration of leave and income compensation differed markedly. Only 20% of those countries replaced 100% of the lost income, with the majority offering 50–75%. Most countries allow a month or more of paid sick leave each year for severe illness, but more than 40 limit payments to less than a month (62).

Most industrialized countries offer the right to paid maternity leave for formal sector employees, but the duration of leave and the nature of the payments also vary substantially. And even though there is a theoretical right to paid maternity leave, few low- and middle-income countries report any financial support for eligible women (Box 1.6).

Financial protection against work incapacity due to illness or pregnancy is generally available only to formal-sector workers. Typically in low-income countries, more than 50% of the working-age population works in the informal sector without access to income replacement at these times (63).

Although this report focuses on financial risk protection linked to the need to pay for health services, this is an important part of broader efforts to ensure social protection in health. As such, WHO is a joint sponsor with the ILO and an active participant in the United Nations initiative to help countries develop comprehensive Social Protection Floors. These include the type of financial risk protection discussed

Box 1.6. Financial risk protection and income replacement: maternity leave

The core element of maternity protection, which guarantees women a period of rest when a child is born (along with the means to support herself and her family and a guarantee of being able to resume work afterwards) is the cash benefit that substitutes the regular income of the mother during a defined period of pregnancy and after childbirth. The cash benefits do not usually replace prior income, but are nonetheless an important social protection measure without which pregnancy and childbirth could pose financial hardships for many families. Maternity leave and the income replacement system that comes with it can also have indirect health consequences; without these measures, women may feel compelled to return to work too quickly after childbirth, before it is medically advisable to do so.

Most industrialized countries allocate considerable resources for maternity leave. In 2007, Norway spent more than any other, allocating US$ 31 000 per baby, per year, for a total US$ 1.8 billion. In contrast most low- and middle-income countries report zero spending on maternal leave, despite the fact that several have enacted legislation guaranteeing it. This may be due to laws going unenforced but may also be explained by the fact that in some countries, maternity leave does not come with any income replacement element.

Source: International Labour Organization.

Making the right choices

There is no single way to develop a financing system to achieve universal coverage. All countries must make choices and trade-offs, particularly in the way that pooled funds are used. It is a constant challenge to balance priorities: funds often remain scarce, yet people demand more and the technologies for improving health are constantly expanding. Such conflicts force policy-makers to make trade-offs in three core areas (Fig. 1.2): the proportion of the population to be covered; the range of services to be made available; and the proportion of the total costs to be met.

The box here labelled "current pooled funds" depicts the situation in a hypothetical country where about half the population is covered for about half the possible services, but where less than half of the cost of these services is met from pooled funds. To get closer to universal coverage, the country would need to extend coverage to more people, offer more services and/or pay a greater part of the cost from pooled funds.

In European countries with long-established social health protection, this "current pooled funds" box fills almost the entire space. But in none of the high-income countries that are commonly said to have achieved universal coverage is 100% of the population covered for 100% of the services that could be made available and for 100% of the cost, with no waiting lists. Each country fills the box in its own way, trading off services and the costs met from pooled funds. Waiting times for services may vary greatly from one country to another, some expensive services might not be provided and citizens may contribute a different proportion of the costs in the form of direct payments.

Nevertheless, everyone in these countries has access to a set of services (prevention, promotion, treatment and rehabilitation) and nearly everyone is protected from severe financial risks thanks to prepayment and pooling of funds. The fundamentals are the same even if the specifics differ, shaped by the expectations of the population and the health providers, the political environment and the availability of funds.

Countries will travel different paths towards universal coverage, depending on where and how they start, and make different choices along the three axes outlined in Fig. 1.2. For example, in settings where all but the elite are currently

Fig. 1.2. **Three dimensions to consider when moving towards universal coverage**

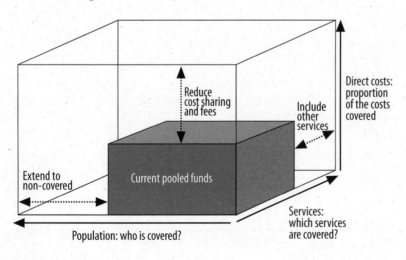

Source: adapted from (*21, 65*).

excluded from health services, moving quickly towards a system that covers everyone, rich or poor, may be a priority, even if the list of services and proportion of costs covered by pooled funds will be relatively small (*21, 66*). Meanwhile, in a broad-based system, with just a few pockets of exclusion, the country may initially opt for a targeted approach, identifying those that are excluded and taking steps to ensure they are covered. In such cases, they can cover more services to the poor and/or cover a higher proportion of the costs.

Many countries setting out on the path to universal coverage begin by targeting groups employed in the so-called formal sector because these groups are more easily identified. But there are downsides to this targeted approach: it can lead to two-tier systems and make conditions worse for those left uncovered; and by achieving partial success, it can slow the impetus for more fundamental reform.

These issues will be taken up in more detail in Chapter 3.

Moving forward

WHO's Constitution describes the fundamental right of every human being to enjoy "the highest attainable standard of health". Universal coverage is the best way to attain that right. It is fundamental to the principle of Health for All set out more than 30 years ago in the Declaration of Alma-Ata. The declaration recognized that promoting and protecting health were also essential to sustained economic and social development, contributing to a better quality of life, social security and peace. The principle of universal coverage was reaffirmed in *The world health report 2008* on primary health care and the subsequent World Health Assembly resolution (*67*), and it was espoused by the 2008 Commission on Social Determinants of Health and the subsequent World Health Assembly resolution on that topic (*68*).

This report reiterates these long-standing beliefs, beliefs that have deepened as countries struggle with their health financing systems. While addressing technical issues related specifically to financing health systems, the report puts fairness and humanity at the heart of the matter. The focus is practical, and optimistic: all countries, at all stages of development, can take steps to move faster towards universal coverage and to maintain their achievements.

In preparing a path towards universal coverage, there are three points to remember.

1. Health systems are "complex adaptive systems" in which relationships are not predictable and components interact in unexpected ways. Participants in the system need to learn and adapt constantly, often in the face of resistance to change (*69*). Even though we offer various routes to universal coverage, countries will need to expect the unexpected.
2. Planning a course towards universal coverage requires countries to first take stock of their current situation. Is there sufficient political and community commitment to achieving and maintaining universal health coverage? This question will mean different things in different contexts but will draw out the prevailing attitudes to social solidarity and self-reliance. A degree of social solidarity is required to develop universal

health coverage, given that any effective system of financial protection for the whole population relies on the readiness of the rich to subsidize the poor, and the healthy to subsidize the sick. Recent research suggests that most, if not all, societies do have a concept of social solidarity when it comes to access to health services and health-care costs, although the nature and extent of these feelings varies across settings (*70*). Put another way, every society has a notion of social justice that puts a limit on how much inequality is acceptable (*71*).

3. Policy-makers then need to decide what proportion of costs will come from pooled funds in the longer run, and how to balance the inevitable tradeoffs in their use – tradeoffs between the proportion of the population, services and costs that can be covered. For those countries focused on maintaining their hard-won gains, continual monitoring and adaptation will be crucial in the face of rapidly developing technologies and changing age structures and disease patterns.

The next three chapters outline practical ways to:

- raise more funds for health where necessary, or maintain funding in the face of competing needs and demands;
- provide or maintain an adequate level of financial risk protection so that people who need services are not deterred from seeking them, and are not subject to catastrophic expenditures or impoverishment for doing so;
- improve efficiency and equity in the way funds are used, effectively ensuring that the available funds go further towards reaching the goal of universal health coverage.

The final chapter outlines practical steps that all countries and international partners can take to raise sufficient funds, achieve optimal pooling and efficiently use the available resources on the path to universal coverage. ∎

References

1. National health accounts [online database]. Geneva, World Health Organization, 2010 (http://www.who.int/nha, accessed 23 June 2010).

2. Preker A et al. Rich-poor differences in health care financing. In: Preker A, Carrin G, eds. *Health financing for poor people: resource mobilization and risk-sharing*. Washington, DC, The World Bank, 2004.

3. Su TT, Kouyaté B, Flessa S. Catastrophic household expenditure for health care in a low-income society: a study from Nouna District, Burkina Faso. *Bulletin of the World Health Organization*, 2006,84:21-27. PMID:16501711

4. Wagstaff A. The economic consequences of health shocks: evidence from Vietnam. *Journal of Health Economics*, 2007,26:82-100. doi:10.1016/j.jhealeco.2006.07.001 PMID:16905205

5. van Doorslaer E et al. Catastrophic payments for health care in Asia. *Health Economics*, 2007,16:1159-1184. doi:10.1002/hec.1209 PMID:17311356

6. Baeza C, Packard T. *Beyond survival: protecting households from health shocks in Latin America*. Washington, DC, The World Bank, 2006.

7. Xu K et al. Protecting households from catastrophic health spending. *Health Aff (Millwood)*, 2007,26:972-983. doi:10.1377/hlthaff.26.4.972 PMID:17630440

8. *Social health protection: an ILO strategy towards universal access to health care*. Geneva, International Labour Organization, 2008 (http://www.ilo.org/public/english/protection/secsoc/downloads/policy/policy1e.pdf, accessed 06 July 2010).

9. Xu K et al. Household catastrophic health expenditure: a multicountry analysis. *Lancet*, 2003,362:111-117. doi:10.1016/S0140-6736(03)13861-5 PMID:12867110

10. Knaul FM et al. [Evidence is good for your health system: policy reform to remedy catastrophic and impoverishing health spending in Mexico]. *Salud Pública de México*, 2007,49:Suppl 1S70-S87. PMID:17469400

11. Yip W, Hsiao WC. Non-evidence-based policy: how effective is China's new cooperative medical scheme in reducing medical impoverishment? *Social Science & Medicine (1982)*, 2009,68:201-209. doi:10.1016/j.socscimed.2008.09.066 PMID:19019519

12. Xu K, Saksena P, Durairaj V. *The drivers of catastrophic expenditure: outpatient services, hospitalization or medicines?* World health report 2010 background paper, no. 21 (http://www.who.int/healthsystems/topics/financing/healthreport/whr_background/en).

13. *World report on disability and rehabilitation*. Geneva, World Health Organization (unpublished).

14. Carrin G, James C, Evans DB. *Achieving universal health coverage: developing the health financing system*. Geneva, World Health Organization, 2005.

15. Resolution WHA58.33. Sustainable health financing, universal coverage and social health insurance In: *Fifty-eighth World Health Assembly, Geneva, 16–25 May 2005* (WHA58/2005/REC/1).

16. *Wading through medical insurance pools: a primer*. The American Academy of Actuaries, 2006 (http://www.actuary.org/pdf/health/pools_sep06.pdf, accessed 06 July 2010).

17. *Annual report 2008*. Ministry of Health, Republic of Rwanda, 2009 (http://www.moh.gov.rw/index.php?option=com_docman&task=doc_download&gid=116&Itemid=14, accessed 06 July 2010).

18. Fernandes Antunes A et al. *Health financing systems review of Rwanda- options for universal coverage*. World Health Organization and Ministry of Health, Republic of Rwanda, 2009.

19. *World health statistics 2010*. Geneva, World Health Organization, 2010.

20. Musango L, Doetinchem O, Carrin G. *De la mutualisation du risque maladie à l'assurance maladie universelle: expérience du Rwanda*. World Health Organization, 2009 (http://www.who.int/health_financing/documents/dp_f_09_01-mutualisation_rwa.pdf, accessed 06 July 2010).

21. *The world health report 2008: primary health care – now more than ever*. Geneva, World Health Organization, 2008.

22. Kalk A et al. Health systems strengthening through insurance subsidies: the GFATM experience in Rwanda. *Tropical medicine & international health : TM & IH*, 2010,15:94-97. PMID:19917038

23. International Health Partnership: a welcome initiative. *Lancet*, 2007,370:801- doi:10.1016/S0140-6736(07)61387-7 PMID:17826149

24. *The International Health Partnership and related initiatives (IHP+)*. (http://www.internationalhealthpartnership.net/en/home, accessed 06 July 2010).

25. Meng Q, Tang S. *Universal coverage of health care in China: challenges and opportunities*. World health report 2010 background paper, no. 7 (http://www.who.int/healthsystems/topics/financing/healthreport/whr_background/en).

26. Barber LS, Yao L. *Health insurance systems in China: a briefing note*. World health report 2010 background paper, no. 37 (http://www.who.int/healthsystems/topics/financing/healthreport/whr_background/en).

27. *Letter to Nancy Pelosi on H.R. 4872, Reconciliation act of 2010 (final health care legislation)*. Washington, DC, Congressional Budget Office, US Congress, 2010 (http://www.cbo.gov/ftpdocs/113xx/doc11379/AmendReconProp.pdf, accessed 07 July 2010).

28. *Focus on health: summary of new health reform law*. Washington, DC, The Henry J. Kaiser Family Foundation, 2010 (http://www.kff.org/healthreform/upload/8061.pdf, accessed 07 July 2010).

29. Missoni E, Solimano G. *Towards universal health coverage: the Chilean experience*. World health report 2010 background paper, no. 4 (http://www.who.int/healthsystems/topics/financing/healthreport/whr_background/en).

30. Whiteford LM, Branch LG. *Primary health care in Cuba: the other revolution*. Lanham, Rowman and Littlefield Publishers, 2008.

31. Rannan-Eliya R, Sikurajapathy L. *Sri Lanka: "Good practice" in expanding health care coverage*. Colombo, Institute for Health Policy, 2008 (Research Studies Series No. 3; http://www.ihp.lk/publications/docs/RSS0903.pdf, accessed 08 July 2010).

32. Damrongplasit K, Melnick GA. Early results from Thailand's 30 Baht Health Reform: something to smile about. *Health Aff (Millwood)*, 2009,28:w457-w466. doi:10.1377/hlthaff.28.3.w457 PMID:19336469

33. Macinko J, Guanais FC, de Fátima M, de Souza M. Evaluation of the impact of the Family Health Program on infant mortality in Brazil, 1990–2002. *Journal of Epidemiology and Community Health*, 2006,60:13-19. doi:10.1136/jech.2005.038323 PMID:16361449

34. Sáenz M, Acosta M, Bermudéz JL. *Universal coverage in Costa Rica: lessons and challenges from a middle-income country.* World health report 2010 background paper, no. 11 (http://www.who.int/healthsystems/topics/financing/healthreport/whr_background/en).

35. D'Almeida S, Durairaj V, Kirigia J. *Ghana's Approach to Social Health Protection.* World health report 2010 background paper, no.2 (http://www.who.int/healthsystems/topics/financing/healthreport/whr_background/en).

36. Kutzin J et al. Bismarck meets Beveridge on the Silk Road: coordinating funding sources to create a universal health financing system in Kyrgyzstan. *Bulletin of the World Health Organization*, 2009,87:549-554. doi:10.2471/BLT.07.049544 PMID:19649370

37. Bayarsaikhan D, Kwon S, Ron A. Development of social health insurance in Mongolia: successes, challenges and lessons. *International Social Security Review*, 2005,58:27-44. doi:10.1111/j.1468-246X.2005.00224.x

38. Jowett M, Shishkin S. *Extending population coverage in the national health insurance scheme in the Republic of Moldova.* Copenhagen, World Health Organization Regional Office for Europe, 2010 (http://www.euro.who.int/__data/assets/pdf_file/0005/79295/E93573.pdf, accessed 06 July 2010).

39. Musango L, Aboubacar I. *Assurance maladie obligatoire au Gabon: un atout pour le bien être de la population.* 2010. World health report 2010 background paper, no.16 (http://www.who.int/healthsystems/topics/financing/healthreport/whr_background/en).

40. Meessen B et al., eds. *Health and social protection: experiences from Cambodia, China and Lao People's Democratic Republic.* Antwerp, ITG Press, 2008.

41. Franco LM et al. Effects of mutual health organizations on use of priority health-care services in urban and rural Mali: a case-control study. *Bulletin of the World Health Organization*, 2008,86:830-838. doi:10.2471/BLT.08.051045 PMID:19030688

42. Jowett M, Hsiao WC. The Philippines: extending coverage beyond the formal sector. In: Hsiao W, Shaw PR, eds. *Social health insurance for developing nations.* Washington, DC, The World Bank, 2007:81–104.

43. Arfa C, Achouri H. Tunisia: good practice in expanding health care coverage. Lessons from reforms in a country in transition. In: Gottret P, Schieber GJ, Waters HR, eds. *Lessons from reforms in low- and middle-income countries. Good practices in health financing.* Washington, DC, The World Bank, 2008:385–437.

44. Axelson H et al. Health financing for the poor produces promising short-term effects on utilization and out-of-pocket expenditure: evidence from Vietnam. *International Journal for Equity in Health*, 2009,8:20-doi:10.1186/1475-9276-8-20 PMID:19473518

45. *OECD Reviews of Health Systems – Turkey.* Organisation for Economic Co-operation and Development and The World Bank, 2008 (http://www.oecd.org/document/60/0,3343,en_2649_33929_42235452_1_1_1_1,00.html, accessed 06 July 2010).

46. Gakidou E et al. Assessing the effect of the 2001–06 Mexican health reform: an interim report card. *Lancet,* 2006,368:1920-1935. PMID:17126725

47. *Health at a glance.* Paris, Organisation for Economic Co-operation and Development, 2009.

48. Carrin G, James C. Social health insurance: key factors affecting the transition towards universal coverage. *International Social Security Review*, 2005,58:45-64. doi:10.1111/j.1468-246X.2005.00209.x

49. Mathauer I et al. *An analysis of the health financing system of the Republic of Korea and options to strengthen health financing performance.* Geneva, World Health Organization, 2009.

50. Jeong H-S. *Expanding insurance coverage to informal sector population: experience from Republic of Korea.* World health report 2010 background paper, no. 38 (http://www.who.int/healthsystems/topics/financing/healthreport/whr_background/en).

51. McIntyre D et al. Beyond fragmentation and towards universal coverage: insights from Ghana, South Africa and the United Republic of Tanzania. *Bulletin of the World Health Organization*, 2008,86:871-876. doi:10.2471/BLT.08.053413 PMID:19030693

52. Himmelstein DU et al. Medical bankruptcy in the United States, 2007: results of a national study. *The American Journal of Medicine*, 2009,122:741-746. doi:10.1016/j.amjmed.2009.04.012 PMID:19501347

53. Emami S. *Consumer overindebtedness and health care costs: how to approach the question from a global perspective.* World health report 2010 background paper, no. 3 (http://www.who.int/healthsystems/topics/financing/healthreport/whr_background/en).

54. Castiglione S. *Compilación de normas en materia de insolvencia por gastos de salud.* World health report 2010 background paper, no. 54 (http://www.who.int/healthsystems/topics/financing/healthreport/whr_background/en).

55. Pradhan M, Prescott N. Social risk management options for medical care in Indonesia. *Health Economics*, 2002,11:431-446. doi:10.1002/hec.689 PMID:12112492

56. Cavagnero E et al. *Health financing in Argentina: an empirical study of health care expenditure and utilization.* Geneva, World Health Organization (Innovations in Health Financing: Working Paper Series, No. 8; http://www.who.int/health_financing/documents/argentina_cavagnero.pdf, accessed 06 July 2010).

57. Houweling TAJ et al. Huge poor-rich inequalities in maternity care: an international comparative study of maternity and child care in developing countries. *Bulletin of the World Health Organization*, 2007,85:745-754. PMID:18038055

58. Xu K, Saksena P, Evans DB. *Health financing and access to effective interventions.* World health report 2010 background paper, no. 8 (http://www.who.int/healthsystems/topics/financing/healthreport/whr_background/en).

59. O'Donnell O et al. Who pays for health care in Asia? *Journal of Health Economics*, 2008,27:460-475. PMID:18179832

60. van Doorslaer E, Masseria C, Koolman X. OECD Health Equity Research GroupInequalities in access to medical care by income in developed countries. *CMAJ : Canadian Medical Association journal = journal de l'Association medicale canadienne*, 2006,174:177-183. doi:10.1503/cmaj.050584 PMID:16415462

61. Das J, Hammer J, Leonard K. The quality of medical advice in low-income countries. *The journal of economic perspectives : a journal of the American Economic Association*, 2008,22:93-114. doi:10.1257/jep.22.2.93 PMID:19768841

62. Scheil-Adlung X, Sandner L. *The case for paid sick leave.* World health report 2010 background paper, no. 9 (http://www.who.int/healthsystems/topics/financing/healthreport/whr_background/en).

63. *World social security report 2010/11. Providing coverage in the time of crisis and beyond.* Geneva, International Labour Organization, 2010.

64. *The social protection floor. A joint crisis initiative of the UN Chief Executives Board for co-ordination on the social protection floor.* Geneva, International Labour Office, and World Health Organization, 2009 (http://www.un.org/ga/second/64/socialprotection.pdf, accessed 8 July 2010).

65. Busse R, Schlette S, eds. *Health Policy Developments Issue 7/8. Focus on prevention, health and aging, new health professions.* Gütersloh, Verlag Bertelsmann Stiftung, 2007 (http://www.hpm.org/Downloads/reports/Health__Policy_Developments_7-8.pdf, accessed 06 July 2010).

66. Houweling TAJ et al. Determinants of under-5 mortality among the poor and the rich: a cross-national analysis of 43 developing countries. *International Journal of Epidemiology*, 2005,34:1257-1265. doi:10.1093/ije/dyi190 PMID:16159940

67. Resolution WHA62.12. Primary health care, including health system strengthening. In: *Sixty-second World Health Assembly, Geneva, 18–27 May 2009.* Geneva, World Health Organization, 2009 (WHA62/2009/REC/1).

68. *Closing the gap in a generation: health equity through action on the social determinants of health. A report of the WHO Commission on Social Determinants of Health.* Geneva, World Health Organization, 2008.

69. *Healthy development: the World Bank strategy for health, nutrition, and population results.* Washington, DC, The World Bank, 2007.

70. James C, Savedoff W. *Risk pooling and redistribution in health care: an empirical analysis of attitudes towards solidarity.* World health report 2010 background paper, no. 5 (http://www.who.int/healthsystems/topics/financing/healthreport/whr_background/en).

71. *Fair society, healthy lives: a strategic review of health inequalities in England post 2010* (http://www.marmotreview.org/AssetLibrary/pdfs/Reports/FairSocietyHealthyLives.pdf, accessed 08 July 2010).

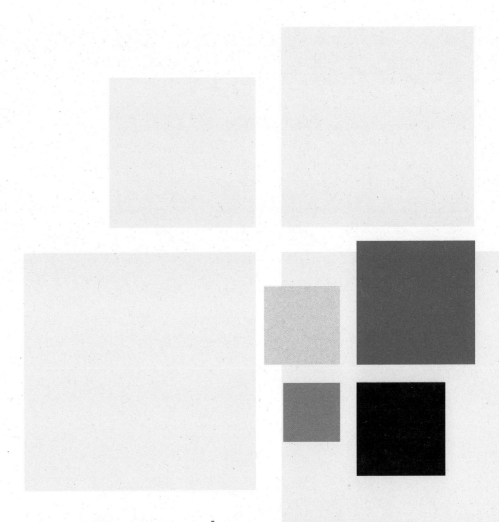

Chapter 2 | More money for health

Key messages

- No country has yet been able to guarantee everyone immediate access to all the services that might maintain or improve their health. They all face resource constraints of one type or another, although these are most critical in low-income countries.

- Every country could raise additional domestic funds for health or diversify their funding sources if they wished to.

- Options include governments giving higher priority to health in their budget allocations, collecting taxes or insurance contributions more efficiently and raising additional funds through various types of innovative financing.

- Taxes on harmful products such as tobacco and alcohol are one such option. They reduce consumption, improve health and increase the resources governments can spend on health.

- Even with these innovations, increased donor flows will be necessary for most of the poorest countries for a considerable period of time. Donor countries can also raise more funds to channel to poorer countries in innovative ways, but they should also do more to meet their stated international commitments for official development assistance (ODA) and to provide more predictable and long-term aid flows.

2

More money for health

Raising resources for health

In 2009, the British National Institute for Health and Clinical Excellence announced that the National Health Service could not offer some expensive medicines for the treatment of renal cancer because they were not cost effective (1). The cuts provoked some public anger (2) but were defended by the institute as being part of difficult but necessary moves to ration resources and set priorities (3). The fact is new medicines and diagnostic and curative technologies become available much faster than new financial resources.

All countries, rich and poor, struggle to raise the funds required to pay for the health services their populations need or demand (which is sometimes a different matter). No country, no matter how rich, is able to provide its entire population with every technology or intervention that may improve health or prolong life. But while rich countries' health systems may face budget limitations – often exacerbated by the dual pressures of ageing populations and shrinking workforces – spending on health remains relatively high. The United States of America and Norway both spend more than US$ 7000 per capita a year; Switzerland more than US$ 6000. Countries from the Organisation for Economic Co-operation and Development (OECD) as a group spend on average about US$ 3600. At the other end of the income scale, some countries struggle to ensure access to even the most basic services: 31 of WHO's Member States spend less than US$ 35 per person per year and four spend less than US$ 10, even when the contributions of external partners are included (4).

But there is scope in all countries to extend financial risk protection and access to health services in a more equitable manner. Rwanda, with per capita national income of about US$ 400, offers a set of basic services to its citizens through a system of health insurances at a cost of just US$ 37 per capita (4). While Rwanda benefits from the financial support of the international donor community, the government also commits 19.5% of its total annual spending to health (4). There are 182 WHO Member States with levels of per capita gross domestic product (GDP) that are comparable with or superior to (in some cases, vastly superior) Rwanda's, and yet many are further away from universal health coverage (4). This needs to change. With few exceptions, countries have no reason to delay improving access to quality health services, while at the same time increasing financial risk protection. This will cost money, and governments need to start thinking about how much is required and where it will come from.

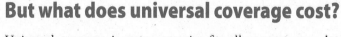

But what does universal coverage cost?

Universal coverage is not a one-size-fits-all concept; nor does coverage for all people necessarily mean coverage for everything. As described in Chapter 1, moving towards universal coverage means working out how best to expand or maintain coverage in three critical dimensions: who is covered from pooled funds; what services are covered; and how much of the cost is covered. Within that broad framework, policy-makers must decide how funds are to be raised and administered.

Thailand offers prescription medicines, ambulatory care, hospitalization, disease prevention and health promotion free of charge to patients, along with more expensive medical services such as radiotherapy and chemotherapy for cancer treatment, surgical operations and critical care for accidents and emergencies. It manages to do all this for just US$ 136 per capita – less than the average health expenditure for lower-middle-income countries, which stands at US$ 153 (4). But Thailand does not cover everything. Until recently it drew the line at renal replacement therapy for end-stage renal disease, for example (Box 2.1). Other countries will draw the line elsewhere.

To know how far you can expand coverage in any of the three dimensions, you must have an idea of what services cost. In 2001 the Commission on Macroeconomics and Health estimated that basic services could be made available for about US$ 34 per person (6), close to what Rwanda is spending now. However, the calculations did not include the full cost of anti-retrovirals or treatment for noncommunicable diseases; nor did they fully take into account investments that might be needed to strengthen a health system so that coverage might be extended to isolated areas.

A more recent estimate of the cost of providing key health services, which was produced by WHO for the high-level Taskforce on Innovative International Financing for Health Systems, suggests that the 49 low-income countries surveyed would need to spend just less than US$ 44 per capita on average (unweighted) in 2009, rising to a little more than US$ 60 per capita by 2015 (7). This estimate includes the cost of expanding health systems so that they can deliver all of the specified mix of interventions. It includes interventions targeting noncommunicable diseases and those for the conditions that are the focus of the health-related

Box 2.1. **Thailand redraws the line in health-care coverage**

When, in 2002, Thailand introduced its universal coverage scheme, which was then called the 30 bhat scheme, it offered comprehensive health care that included not just basics, but services such as radiotherapy, surgery and critical care for accidents and emergencies. It did not, however, cover renal-replacement therapy. "There was a concern that [renal-replacement therapy] could burden the system as major health risks leading to kidney diseases, such as diabetes and hypertension, were still not well controlled," says Dr Prateep Dhanakijcharoen, deputy secretary general of the National Health Security Office that administers the scheme. Renal replacement therapy is expensive; haemodialysis costs about 400 000 baht (US$ 12 000) per patient, per year in Thailand, four times higher than the 100 000-baht per quality-adjusted life year threshold set by the security office's benefit package subcommittee for medicines and treatments within the scheme.

That said, Dhanakijcharoen believes the scheme should have covered kidney disease from the outset. This view is shared by Dr Viroj Tangcharoensathien, director of the International Health Policy Programme at the Ministry of Public Health. For Tangcharoensathien, it was simply a matter of fairness: "There are three health-care schemes in Thailand," he says. "Only the scheme did not include renal-replacement therapy. Meanwhile, half of those people in the scheme are in the poorest quintile of the Thai economy." His sense of injustice was shared by other people, such as Subil Noksakul, a 60-year-old patient who spent his life-savings on renal replacement therapy over a period of 19 years. "I once managed to save seven million baht," he says, "but my savings are now all gone." In 2006 Noksakul founded the Thai Kidney Club, which has raised kidney patients' awareness of their rights and put pressure on the National Health Security Office to provide treatment. Finally, in October 2008, the then public health minister, Mongkol Na Songkhla, included renal-replacement therapy in the scheme.

Source: Excerpt from (5).

Millennium Development Goals (MDGs). These figures, however, are simply an (unweighted) average across the 49 countries at the two points in time. Actual needs will vary by country: five of the countries in that study will need to spend more than US$ 80 per capita in 2015, while six will need to spend less than US$ 40[a].

This does not mean that the 31 countries spending less than US$ 35 per person on health should abandon efforts to raise resources to move closer to universal health coverage. But they will need to tailor their expansion according to their resources. It also means that although it is within their capacity to raise additional funds domestically – as we show in the next two sections – for the immediate future they will also require external help. Even with relatively high levels of domestic growth, and national budgets that prioritize health, only eight of the 49 countries have any chance of financing the required level of services from domestic resources in 2015 (7).

Many richer countries will also need to raise additional funds to meet constantly evolving health demands, driven partly by ageing populations and the new medicines, procedures and technologies being developed to serve them. A key aspect of this complex issue is the diminishing working-age population in some countries. Dwindling contributions from income taxes or wage-based health insurance deductions (payroll taxes) will force policy-makers to consider alternative sources of funding.

Broadly speaking, there are three ways to raise additional funds or diversify sources of funding: the first is to make health a higher priority in existing spending, particularly in a government's budget; the second is to find new or diversified sources of domestic funding; and the third is to increase external financial support. We review these options in turn, the first two being important for countries at all stages of development, rich or poor. The chapter concludes by considering development assistance for health for low- and middle-income countries.

Ensuring a fair share of total government spending on health

Even in countries where external assistance is important, its contribution is generally much less than the money for health collected domestically. In the low-income countries, for example, the average (unweighted) contribution from external sources in 2007 was a little less than 25% of total health expenditure, the rest coming from domestic sources (4). It is critical, therefore, to sustain and, where necessary, increase domestic resources for health, even in the poorest countries (8). This is just as important in higher-income settings.

Governments finance health improvements both directly, through investments in the health sector, and indirectly, through spending on social determinants – by reducing poverty or improving female education levels, for example. Although it captures only the direct component, the proportion of overall spending allocated to the health sector provides important insights into the value that governments place on health, something that varies greatly between countries. Fig. 2.1 shows the average share of government spending

Fig. 2.1. Government expenditure on health as a percentage of total government expenditures by WHO region, 2000–2007[a]

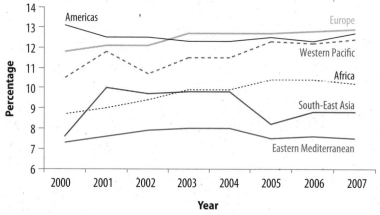

^a These are unweighted averages. Government health expenditure includes health spending by all government ministries and all levels of government. It also includes spending from compulsory social health insurance contributions.
Source: (4).

on health by WHO region for the period from 2000 to 2007, the last year for which figures are available. The figures include contributions from external partners channelled through government budgets in both the numerator and denominator because few countries report them separately.

Governments in the Americas, the European and Western Pacific Regions, on average, allocate more to health than the other regions. African countries as a group are increasing their commitment to health as are those in the European and Western Pacific Regions. In South-East Asia, the relative priority given to health fell in 2004–2005, but is increasing again, while governments in the WHO Eastern Mediterranean Region have reduced the share allocated to health since 2003.

Some of the variation across regions can be explained by differences in country wealth. Generally, health accounts for a higher proportion of total government spending as countries get richer. Chile is a good example, having increased its share of government spending on health from 11% in 1996 to 16% a decade later during a period of strong economic growth (9).

But a country's relative wealth is not the only factor at play. Substantial variations across countries with similar income levels indicate different levels of government commitment to health. This can be illustrated in many ways, but here we cite the WHO Regional Office for Europe, which has countries at all income levels. In Fig. 2.2, the vertical axis shows the proportion of total government spending allocated to health, and the bars on the horizontal axis represent countries in that region, ordered from lowest to highest levels of GDP per capita.

Budget allocations to health in the WHO European Region vary from a low 4% of total government spending to almost 20%. Importantly, even though the priority given to health in overall government budgets generally increases with national income, some governments choose to allocate a high proportion of their total spending to health despite relatively low levels of national income; others that are relatively rich allocate lower proportions to health.

This pattern can also be seen globally. Although government commitments to health tend to increase with higher levels of national income, some low-income countries allocate higher proportions of total government spending to health than their high-income counterparts; 22 low-income countries across the world allocated more than 10% to health in 2007 while, on the other hand, 11 high-income countries allocated less than 10%.

While the African Region does not post the lowest result in Fig. 2.1, the relatively low level of domestic investment in health in some of its countries

is cause for concern because it is in sub-Saharan Africa that the slowest progress has been made towards the MDGs (*10*, *11*). In 2007, only three African countries – Liberia, Rwanda and the United Republic of Tanzania – had followed through on the 2001 Abuja Declaration, in which African leaders pledged to "set a target of allocating at least 15% of their annual budgets to the improvement of the health sector" (*12*). Disappointingly, 19 African countries in 2007 allocated a lower proportion of their total government budgets to health than they did before Abuja (*4*).

Governments have, therefore, the option to re-examine budget priorities with health in mind. Although funding needs vary with differences in costs, population age structures and patterns of disease, many governments of rich and poor countries could allocate much more to health from available resources. The gains could be substantial. Taken as a group, the low-income countries could raise (at least) an additional US$ 15 billion dollars per year for health from domestic sources by increasing the share of health in total government spending (net of external aid inflows) to 15%. For the same countries, the increased funding for the period 2009–2015 would be about US$ 87 billion (*7*).

There are several reasons countries do not prioritize health in their budgets, some fiscal, some political, some perhaps linked to the perception in ministries of finance that ministries of health are not efficient. In addition, the budget priority governments give to health reflects the degree to which those in power care, or are made to care, about the health of their people. Dealing with universal health coverage also means dealing with the poor and the marginalized, people who are often politically disenfranchised and lack representation.

This is why making health a key political issue is so important and why civil society, joined by eminent champions of universal coverage, can help persuade politicians to move health financing for universal coverage to the top of the political agenda (*13*). Improving efficiency and accountability may also convince ministries of finance, and increasingly donors, that more funding will be well used (we will return to this in Chapter 4).

Learning the language of economists and the type of arguments that convince them of the need for additional funding can also help ministries of health negotiate with a ministry of finance. It also helps them understand the complexities of changes in the way health is funded and then to take the opportunities that arise. For example, it is important that ministries of health

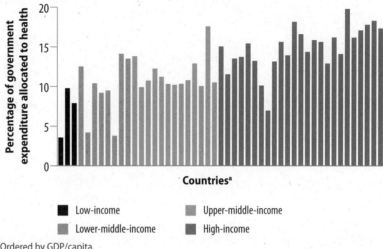

Fig. 2.2. **The share of total government expenditure allocated to health in the WHO European Region, 2007**

Percentage of government expenditure allocated to health

Countries[a]

■ Low-income
■ Lower-middle-income
■ Upper-middle-income
■ High-income

[a] Ordered by GDP/capita.
Source: (*4*).

keep track of negotiations between donors and ministries of finance relating to debt relief and general budget support (*14–16*). They need not only to understand these processes but also be able to discuss and negotiate with the minister of finance for a share of available funds.

Diversifying domestic sources of revenue

There are two main ways to increase domestic funding for health: one is to allocate more of the existing financial resources to health, as discussed in the previous section; the other is to find new methods to raise funds or to diversify the sources.

Collecting taxes and insurance contributions more efficiently would effectively raise additional funds. Improving revenue collection is something that all countries might need to consider, though this may be problematic for many lower-income countries with large informal sectors (*17*). This does not mean, however, that it cannot be done. Though a complex and often daunting task, there have been improvements in tax collection in several settings, including countries where there is a large informal sector, Indonesia being a notable example (Box 2.2).

The type of reform undertaken by Indonesia requires investment and a level of technology and infrastructure beyond the scope of some countries. It also requires improving tax collection from corporations, not just individuals. This can again be problematic in low-income countries that host extractive industries. Low compliance by just a few large potential taxpayers can lead to considerable revenue loss.

Increasing globalization and the location of corporate assets offshore – often in tax havens –raises the potential for lost tax revenue, either through unintended legal loopholes or through the illegal use of hidden accounts by individuals. All OECD countries now accept Article 26 of the OECD model tax convention, covering the exchange of information, and more than 360 tax information exchange agreements have been signed (*19*). It is hoped that global corporations and the financial institutions that service them will be more transparent in their dealings in the future, and that the countries hosting them will get a fairer share of tax receipts, some of which, hopefully, will go into paying for health.

But tax compliance can also be fostered when citizens believe they are getting a good deal from governments. A 2009 study concluded that while the threat of detection and punishment was a key factor in compliance, perceptions of

---

Box 2.2. Indonesia increases tax revenues by encouraging compliance

Even before the 1997–1998 Asian crisis, non-oil tax collection in Indonesia was on the decline, reaching a low of 9.6% of GDP in 2000. The tax policy regime was complicated and tax administration weak. At the end of 2001, the Directorate General of Taxation (DGT) decided to simplify the tax system and its administration. The aim was to encourage voluntary compliance, whereby taxpayers would self-assess, then pay the tax on income declared. Voluntary compliance typically makes up 90% of total tax revenue for a country and represents a line of least resistance for governments seeking to enhance tax yields. In contrast, enforced collection tends to be arduous, labour and capital intensive, and yields relatively little return.

The DGT drafted tax laws and regulations that were clear, accessible and consistently applied, and adopted a policy of zero-tolerance towards corruption. The DGT also introduced procedures to resolve disputes quickly, cheaply and impartially, and encouraged transparency by making all actions taken by the tax administration subject to public scrutiny. Performance and efficiency were improved partly by digitizing a previously paper-based process. Positive results followed, with the tax yield rising from 9.9% to 11% of non-oil GDP in the four years after implementation. The additional tax revenues meant that overall government spending could be increased; health spending rose faster than other.

Source: (*18*).

the quality of governance were also important (*20*). Compliance was notably higher in Botswana, where government services were perceived to be good, and lower in some neighbouring countries where the quality of government services was perceived to be lower.

In the short-term, low-income countries with large informal economies will tend to focus on taxes that are relatively easy to collect, such as those on formal-sector employees and corporations, import or export duties of various types and value added tax (VAT) (*21*). Ghana, for example, meets 70–75% of funding needs for its National Health Insurance Scheme with general tax funding, notably through a 2.5% national health insurance levy on VAT, which stands at 12.5%. The rest of the funding comes from other public funds and development partners, while premiums, the traditional revenue source for insurance, account for only 3% of total income. The VAT-based National Health Insurance Scheme has been able to support an increase in total health expenditure through domestically generated pooled funds. At the same time it has lessened the system's dependence on direct payments such as user fees as a source of finance (*22*).

Chile, an upper-middle-income country, in 2003 also introduced a 1% increase in VAT to fund health. Even richer countries are being forced to diversify their sources of financing, away from the traditional forms of income tax and wage-based insurance deductions. An ageing population means a lower proportion of people in work and wage-based contributions no longer cover the full costs of health care. Germany, for example, has recently started to inject money from general tax revenues into the social health insurance system through a new central fund called the *Gesundheitsfond*. The French national health insurance scheme has been partly funded for 30 years by the *Contribution sociale généralisée*, which includes taxes levied on real estate and capital gains in addition to more traditional forms of revenue such as income taxes (*23*).

Exploring sources of domestic financing for health

The international community has taken several important steps since 2000 to raise additional funding to improve health in poor countries. They are outlined briefly here because they offer ideas for countries to raise domestic funds as well.

One of the earliest steps was the air-ticket levy used to fund Unitaid, a global drug-purchase facility for HIV/AIDS, tuberculosis and malaria (*24, 25*). It has provided almost US$ 1 billion to date, which, when combined with more traditional development assistance, has allowed Unitaid to finance projects in 93 countries, totalling US$ 1.3 billion since 2006 (*26*). At the same time, the buying power of Unitaid has resulted in significant falls in the prices of certain products, increasing the quantities that are available to improve health. More recently, the Millennium Foundation on Innovative Financing for Health launched a voluntary solidarity levy under the name MassiveGood, whereby individuals can complement Unitaid funding through voluntary contributions when they buy travel and tourism products (*27, 28*).

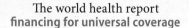

The sale of bonds guaranteed by donor countries and issued on international capital markets is estimated to have raised more than US$ 2 billion since 2006 (*29*). These funds are channelled to the International Financing Facility for Vaccines, linked to the GAVI Alliance. The governments of eight countries have pledged the funds necessary to repay these bonds when they mature, although whether this mechanism results in additional resources being raised for global health depends critically on whether the repayments are considered a part of the planned future aid disbursements or are additional to them. At the minimum, however, they allow aid to be disbursed immediately, not deferred.

More recently, the high-level Taskforce on Innovative International Financing for Health Systems reviewed a wider range of options for supplementing traditional bilateral funding for aid (*30*). The taskforce concluded that a currency transaction levy had the potential to raise the greatest amount of money globally: an annual sum in excess of US$ 33 billion, but recommended several additional options as well (*30, 31*).

These developments have helped pinpoint new sources of funds and maintained the momentum for increased international solidarity in health financing. However, discussions on innovative financing have so far ignored the needs of countries to find new sources of domestic funds for their own use: low- and middle-income countries that simply need to raise more and high-income countries that need to innovate in the face of changing health needs, demands and work patterns.

To help this discussion, a list of options for countries seeking to increase or diversify domestic sources of funding is provided in Table 2.1, drawing on the work cited above. Not all the options will be applicable in all settings, and the income-generating potential of those that are will also vary by country, though we do make some suggestions about the likely level of funding that could be raised at the country level. For example, even though the currency transactions levy proposed by the high-level taskforce has the potential to raise large sums of money, the financial transactions and products that it would be based on are concentrated in higher-income countries. Indeed, 10 high-income countries account for 85% of the traditional foreign exchange trade (*35*). Trading volumes are light in most low- and middle-income countries, so this specific levy may not apply to most of them. There are some exceptions: India has a significant foreign exchange market, with daily turnover of US$ 34 billion (*35*). A currency transaction levy of 0.005% on this volume of trade might yield India about US$ 370 million per year if it chose to implement it.

So-called solidarity taxes on specific goods and services are another promising option, offering a proven capacity to generate income, relatively low administration costs and sustainability. With political support, they can be implemented quickly. The mandatory solidarity levy on airline tickets, for example, might require 2–12 months for implementation (*30*).

Introducing mechanisms that involve taxes can be politically sensitive and will invariably be resisted by particular interest groups. A tax on foreign exchange transactions, for example, may be perceived as a brake on the banking sector or as a disincentive to exporters/importers. When Gabon introduced a tax on money transfers in 2009 to raise funds to subsidize health care for low-income groups, some people protested that it constituted

Table 2.1.   **Domestic options for innovative financing**

Options	Fund-raising potential[a]	Assumptions/examples	Remarks
Special levy on large and profitable companies – a tax/levy that is imposed on some of the big economic companies in the country	$$–$$$	Australia has recently imposed a levy on mining companies; Gabon has introduced a levy on mobile phone companies; Pakistan has a long-standing tax on pharmaceutical companies	Context specific
Levy on currency transactions – a tax on foreign exchange transactions in the currency markets	$$–$$$	Some middle-income countries with important currency transaction markets could raise substantial new resources	Might need to be coordinated with other financial markets if undertaken on a large scale
Diaspora bonds – government bonds for sale to nationals living abroad	$$	Lowers the cost of borrowing for the country (patriotic discount); have been used in India, Israel and Sri Lanka, although not necessarily for health	For countries with a significant out-of-country population
Financial transaction tax – a levy on all bank account transactions or on remittance transactions	$$	In Brazil there was a bank tax in the 1990s on bank transactions, although it was subsequently replaced by a tax on capital flows to/from the country; Gabon has implemented a levy on remittance transactions	There seems to have been stronger opposition from interest groups to this tax than others (32)
Mobile phone voluntary solidarity contribution – solidarity contributions would allow individuals and corporations to make voluntary donations via their monthly mobile phone bill	$$	The global market for postpaid mobile phone services is US$ 750 billion, so even taking 1% of that would raise a lot of money; relevant to low-, middle- and high-income countries (33)	Establishment and running costs could be about 1–3% of revenues (33)
Tobacco excise tax – an excise tax on tobacco products **Alcohol excise tax** – an excise tax on alcohol products	$$	These excise taxes on tobacco and alcohol exist in most countries but there is ample scope to raise them in many without causing a fall in revenues	Reduces tobacco and alcohol consumption, which has a positive public health impact
Excise tax on unhealthy food (sugar, salt) – an excise tax on unhealthy foodstuffs and ingredients	$–$$	Romania is proposing to implement a 20% levy on foods high in fat, salt, additives and sugar (34)	Reduces consumption of harmful foods and improves health
Selling franchised products or services – similar to the Global Fund's ProductRED, whereby companies are licensed to sell products and a proportion of the profits goes to health	$	Selling franchised products or services from which a percentage of the profits goes to health	Such a scheme could operate in low- and middle-income countries in ways that did not compete with the Global Fund
Tourism tax – a tourism tax would be levied on activities linked largely to international visitors	$	Airport departure taxes are already widely accepted; a component for health could be added, or levies found	The gain would vary greatly between countries depending on the strength of their tourism sector

[a] $, low fund-raising potential; $$, medium fund-raising potential; $$$, high fund-raising potential.

Box 2.3. To hypothecate or not to hypothecate?

Hypothecated taxes, sometimes called earmarked taxes, are those designated for a particular programme or use. Examples include TV licence fees that are used to fund public broadcasting and road tolls that are used to maintain and upgrade roads. The Western Australian Health Promotion Foundation's Healthway was created in 1991 on this basis, funded initially out of an increased levy on tobacco products, while the Republic of Korea instituted a National Health Promotion Fund in 1995 funded partly from tobacco taxes (40). The Thai Health Promotion Fund, established in 2001, was financed with a 2% additional surcharge on tobacco and alcohol (41, 42).

Ministries of health are often in favour of these taxes because they guarantee funding, particularly for health promotion and prevention. It is difficult for these activities to compete with curative services for funding, partly because they are perceived to be less urgent, and partly because they tend to yield results over the longer term, making them less attractive to politicians with an eye on the electoral cycle or to insurance funds interested in financial viability.

Ministries of finance, however, rarely endorse hypothecation because they feel that it undermines their mandate to allocate budgets. By taking decisions on spending away from government, hypothecating tax revenues can constrain the government's ability to deal with economic cycles.

In practice, hypothecating any particular form of tax – e.g. a tobacco tax – for health does not guarantee that overall government funding to health will increase. Most government revenues are essentially fungible; an increase in health funding from hypothecated taxes may be offset by a reduction in flows from the rest of the budget. So whether hypothecation leads to a net increase in funding for health, or for a particular activity, is an empirical question.

A pragmatic approach is likely to pay higher dividends for health than insisting on hypothecation. If governments can be persuaded to allocate any of the new funding sources discussed in this chapter to health, in their entirety, so much the better. If they cannot, there is still likely to be an increase in health funding because health usually gets a share of any increase in government spending. Though this increase might be lower than in the case of hypothecation, health advocates need to be sure that insisting on hypothecation does not result in a ministry of finance opposing the new tax totally, so that no new monies at all are received.

Source (43).

an exchange restriction. Gabon nevertheless imposed a 1.5% levy on the post-tax profits of companies that handle remittances and a 10% tax on mobile phone operators. Between them, the two taxes raised the equivalent of US$ 30 million for health in 2009 (36, 37). Similarly, the Pakistan government has been taxing the profits of pharmaceutical companies to finance part of its health spending for many years (38).

Meanwhile, so-called sin taxes have the advantage of raising funds and improving health at the same time by reducing consumption of harmful products such as tobacco or alcohol. Studies in 80 countries have found that the real price of tobacco, adjusted for purchasing power, fell between 1990 and 2000. Although there have been some increases since 2000, there is great scope for revenue raising in this area, as advocated by the WHO Framework Convention on Tobacco Control (39).

It is not possible in this report to provide estimates of how much money could be raised by each of these innovative financing mechanisms on a country-by-country basis. But WHO has analysed the potential gains from increasing taxes on tobacco in 22 of the 49 low-income countries for which sufficient data to make the calculations are available. Excise taxes in these countries range from 11% to 52% of the retail price of the most popular brand of cigarettes, representing a nominal range of US$ 0.03–0.51 per pack of 20 (37). We estimate that a 50% increase in excise taxes would generate US$ 1.42 billion in additional funds for these countries – quite a substantial sum. In countries like the Lao People's Democratic Republic, Madagascar and Viet Nam, the extra revenue would represent a 10% increase or more in total health expenditure, and a more than 25% increase in the government's health budget, assuming the revenue raised was fully allocated to health (Box 2.3). Viewed another way, this simple measure could raise additional funding that would more than double the current levels of external aid to health in certain countries.

There is increasing international concern about the adverse health and economic consequences of alcohol consumption, and pricing policies can be at the core of strategies to address these concerns. For example, in Moscow, alcohol prices were increased by 20% in August 1985 and another 25% the following year. The result was a dramatic fall (28.6%) in alcohol consumption over the next 18 months. Hospital admissions for alcohol-related mental and behavioural disorders and deaths from liver cirrhosis, alcohol poisoning and other violence decreased substantially. These measures ended in 1987 and in the subsequent period, when alcohol prices grew at a much slower rate than other prices, many of these positive trends were reversed (44).

Analysis of selected countries for which data are available on the consumption, taxation and pricing of alcoholic beverages shows that, if excise taxes were raised to at least 40% of the retail price, substantial additional revenue could be generated and the harmful effects of drinking alcohol reduced. For the 12 low-income countries in the sample, consumption levels would fall by more than 10%, while tax revenues would more than triple to a level amounting to 38% of total health spending in those countries (37).

These sums are not negligible. If all countries chose just one of the options described in Table 2.1 and also gave higher priority to health in government budgets, substantial additional amounts could be raised for health.

External financial assistance

Prior to the global economic downturn that started late in 2008, development assistance for health from richer to poorer countries was increasing at a robust rate. Low-income countries saw funding from external sources rise on average from 16.5% of their total health expenditures in 2000 to 24.8% in 2007 (4). According to the databases maintained by the OECD's development assistance committee, government commitments for health reported by bilateral donors jumped from about US$ 4 billion in 1995 to US$ 17 billion in 2007 and US$ 20 billion in 2008[a].

This may represent a significant underestimate given that the committee database does not capture all contributions from non-OECD governments, such as China, India and some Middle-Eastern countries; reports data for only a limited number of multilateral institutions; and does not collate funds provided by key private players in the health domain such as the Bill & Melinda Gates Foundation, other private foundations, and nongovernmental organizations. A recent study suggested that the combined contribution from all these sources might have been about US$ 21.8 billion, almost US$ 5 billion greater than reported to the OECD in 2007 (45).

However, in at least four key ways, the outlook for aid-recipient countries is less positive than these numbers might suggest.

First, despite the increase in external support, total health expenditures remain pitifully low – insufficient to ensure universal access to even a basic set of health services in many countries. We reported earlier that only eight of the 49 low-income countries included in the analysis for the high-level taskforce had any prospect of raising all of the resources required to meet the health goals of the Millennium Declaration from domestic sources by 2015. The other countries would require additional inputs from external sources ranging from US$ 2 to US$ 41 per capita in 2015.

Second, even though external funding has increased substantially, about half of the countries reporting their development assistance disbursements to OECD are on track to meet the targets they have committed to internationally (for overall development, including health) (46). The other countries are failing to meet their pledges, some by a long way. Slow progress towards fulfilling these commitments comes at a huge human cost; three million additional lives could be saved before 2015 if all donors met their promises (7).

Third, the development assistance for health numbers reported above represent commitments; actual disbursements are lower. In addition, some of the funds that donors report as disbursed do not arrive in recipient countries for them to spend. A sometimes considerable proportion of aid is devoted to so-called technical cooperation. This was the case between 2002 and 2006, for example, when the committee database reported that more than 40% of health official development assistance (ODA)[b] was absorbed by technical support, often funding nationals of the donor country to provide assistance or training to recipient countries (47). While technical support might be useful, reported disbursements overstate the availability of funds that recipient countries can use to improve health locally.

Finally, concerns have also been expressed recently that some of the aid arriving in countries is subject to spending constraints. Macroeconomic and monetary targets set for inflation and the level of foreign exchange reserves are based on a concept of prudent macroeconomic management. Some say this prevents the disbursed aid being fully exploited because a portion of the aid that arrives in the country is believed to be withheld from circulation to avoid inflation, or is used to build up foreign exchange reserves (48–50).

There is currently vigorous debate about whether the targets for inflation and foreign exchange reserves set in countries are too stringent and restrict them from spending the aid that donors provide for health and development (39, 51, 52). Moreover, it is not yet clear how much additional spending might become available if macroeconomic targets were relaxed; recent work suggests that the additional spending would probably be small when compared with the extra funds that would flow from governments giving a higher priority to health when allocating their own budgets (53).

Re-examining the targets for macroeconomic prudence is, perhaps, one option for increasing the amount of aid that can be spent. Deficit spending is another. Countries can either borrow so that they can spend now, or perform what has been recently called quantitative easing – printing money to finance current spending. Neither is a viable long-term strategy because debt incurred now will have to be paid back, while printing money will increase inflationary pressures at some point.

A more sustainable option is for external partners to reduce the volatility of their aid flows. This would, at a minimum, allow government budget ceilings in health to be relaxed and more aid could be used to improve health. A more ambitious agenda has recently been proposed whereby donor and recipient countries would review the entire aid architecture and its governance (54, 55). The objective would be to move away from viewing aid as a charity, at the total discretion of donors, towards a system of mutual global responsibility that would enable more predictable, probably larger flows of funding to populations that need it.

Effect of economic downturn on development assistance

Precisely what effect the financial and economic downturn that started in 2008 will have on development assistance for health is still unclear. However, there are concerns that the downturn may act as a brake at time when there is growing global acceptance that external financial support for health needs to rise.

Overall bilateral development assistance tends to reflect economic growth in the donor country. This does not always hold true for development assistance for health, which in some recent economic crises has been insulated, despite overall development assistance falling (56). However, many governments that have traditionally been major bilateral contributors of development assistance for health are now burdened with considerably more debt than they carried in past downturns, much of it incurred to soften the effects of the economic crisis and stimulate growth in their own countries. Some of those governments are now trying to reduce their debt with spending cuts.

The OECD reports that while some donors are promising to maintain their commitments to ODA for 2010, some large donors have already reduced or postponed their pledges (46). Overall ODA is still expected to grow in 2010 but at a lower rate than initially forecast. This is not good news, and it is to be hoped that the major donors will not only maintain their current levels of assistance to poorer countries but also increase them to the extent necessary to fulfil their international aid promises. Similarly, it is hoped that they will not respond to high levels of government indebtedness by cutting domestic health services in their own countries.

Even before the current global economic downturn, there was cause for concern about the way health aid funding moves around the globe. The channelling of aid into high-profile health initiatives while others are neglected is one such concern. Between 2002 and 2006, financial commitments to low-income countries focused on MDG 6 (combat HIV/AIDS, malaria and other diseases, including tuberculosis), which accounted for 46.8% of total external assistance for health. It has been estimated that this left only US$ 2.25 per capita per year for everything else – child and maternal health (MDGs 4 and 5), nutrition (MDG 1), noncommunicable diseases and strengthening health systems (47). The money required to strengthen health systems alone exceeds this figure – US$ 2.80 per capita is needed each year to train additional health workers, and this amount does not even include the funding necessary to pay their salaries (57).

The picture is less bleak if we take into account recent efforts by the GAVI Alliance and the Global Fund to Fight AIDS, Tuberculosis and Malaria to support health systems development and capacity-building. Nevertheless, diseases outside these headline issues continue to be neglected by donors, as do health systems issues such as management, logistics, procurement, infrastructure and workforce development (58).

The imbalance in aid allocation is apparent also when broken down by country; some countries are particularly well funded while others receive virtually nothing. Fig. 2.3 shows that the recipient countries receiving more than US$ 20 per capita in external assistance for health in 2007 were middle-income countries, while the bulk of the low-income countries received less than US$ 5 per capita. Many of the poorest countries receive substantially less development assistance for health than their much richer neighbours. For example, Namibia, a lower-middle-income country, received about US$ 34 per capita for health in 2007, compared with US$ 10 in Mozambique, US$ 4.40 in the Democratic Republic of the Congo and US$ 2.80 in the Republic of Guinea (4). It would appear that many other factors, in addition to need, determine aid allocations.

The high-level taskforce suggested that the focus of many external partners on a few high-profile programmes and countries ran counter to the spirit of the 2005 Paris Declaration on Aid Effectiveness, which seeks to enable recipient countries to formulate and execute their own national plans according to their own national priorities (59). In its report, the taskforce called for a shift away from "international financing mechanisms that build on project applications approved in a development partner's global headquarters or capital" (60). What is required is a refocusing on agreed financial contributions to national health plans rather than a continuation of project-based aid. We are yet to see the impact of these ideals reflected in official figures. According to a study prepared for the Norwegian Agency for Development Cooperation, between 2002 and 2007 the number of health-related projects, rather than falling, doubled to 20 000. Most of these were small, with an average disbursement of only US$ 550 000 (61). The need to manage, monitor and report on a multitude of small projects imposes high transaction costs on the recipient country.

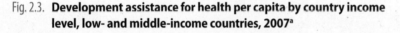

Fig. 2.3. **Development assistance for health per capita by country income level, low- and middle-income countries, 2007**[a]

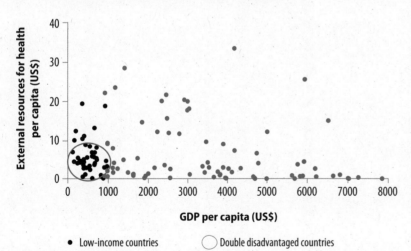

- Low-income countries
- Middle-income countries
- ◯ Double disadvantaged countries

[a] Excluding small island states.
Source: World Health Organization national health accounts series (4).

The Paris Declaration also emphasized that funding should be predictable and long-term. When countries cannot rely on steady funding – in Burkina Faso, per capita development assistance for health fluctuated from US$ 4 to US$ 10 and back down to US$ 8 between 2003 and 2006 – it is virtually impossible to plan for the future. A few low-income countries have two thirds of their total health expenditure funded by external resources, making the predictability of aid flows a critical concern for them (4, 62).

Some development partners are already starting to depart from traditional short-term ODA commitments in the way they structure their contributions. European Union MDG contracts are an example, offering flexible, performance-based budget support over a period of six years. Not everyone likes this kind of commitment because it ties up future aid budgets. That said, in the Accra Agenda for Action of 2008, OECD development assistance committee donors committed to providing recipient countries with information on their "rolling three- to five-year expenditure and/ or implementation plans" – the beginning perhaps of longer-term commitments (*59*).

Conclusion

Countries need to adapt their financing systems continually to raise sufficient funds for their health systems. Many high-income countries are facing a decline in the proportion of their working-age population and having to consider alternatives to traditional sources of revenue in the form of income taxes and health insurance contributions from workers and their employers. In many lower-income countries, more people work in the informal than the formal sector, making it difficult to collect income taxes and wage-based health insurance contributions.

There are several options for raising additional funds for health, a list of which is provided in Table 2.1. Not all will apply to all countries, and the income-generating potential and political feasibility of those that do will vary by country. In some cases, however, the additional income to be derived from any one or more of these options could be substantial, possibly much more than current aid inflows. These innovative and additional mechanisms are not, however, the only option. Many governments, in rich and poor countries, still give a relatively low priority to health when allocating funds. It is important, therefore, to better equip the ministries of health to negotiate with ministries of finance and planning, as well as with international financial institutions. But the message of this chapter is that every country could do more domestically to raise additional funds for health.

Innovative financing should not be seen, however, as a substitute for ODA flows from donor nations. Calls for recipient countries to use external funds more transparently and efficiently are understandable. But such concerns should not stop richer countries keeping the promises they have made in Paris and Accra. Collective action that has led to the International Financing Facility for Immunization and to the Millennium Foundation has been invaluable in financing global public goods for health, but there is no need for countries to wait for more global collaboration before acting. If the governments of donor countries kept their current international aid promises, allocating funds in ways that supported country-led national health plans, the international community would already be well advanced towards meeting the 2015 MDGs. If, in addition, each donor country adopted just one of the innovative options described here and used the revenue to supplement ODA, they would be laying the foundations for sustained movement towards universal health coverage and improved health into the future. ∎

References

1. *NICE draft recommendation on the use of drugs for renal cancer.* National Institute for Health and Clinical Excellence, 2009 (http://www.nice.org.uk/newsroom/pressreleases/pressreleasearchive/PressReleases2009.jsp?domedia =1&mid=42007069-19B9-E0B5-D429BEDD12DFE74E, accessed 3 April 2010).

2. Kidney cancer patients denied life-saving drugs by NHS rationing body NICE. *Daily Mail,* 29 April 2009 (http://www.dailymail.co.uk/health/article-1174592/Kidney-cancer-patients-denied-life-saving-drugs-NHS-rationing-body-NICE.html, accessed 3 April 2010).

3. *NICE issues guidance on the use of other treatment options for renal cancer.* National Institute for Health and Clinical Excellence, 2009 (http://www.nice.org.uk/newsroom/pressreleases/pressreleasearchive/PressReleases2009.jsp?domedia=1&mid=4BAE772C-19B9-E0B5-D449E739CDCD7772, accessed 7 July 2010).

4. National Health Accounts [online database]. Geneva, World Health Organization (http://www.who.int/nha, accessed 4 May 2010).

5.. Treerutkuarkul A, Treerutkuarkul A. Thailand: health care for all, at a price. *Bulletin of the World Health Organization,* 2010,88:84-85. doi:10.2471/BLT.10.010210 PMID:20428360

6. *Macroeconomics and health: investing in health for economic development.* Geneva, World Health Organization, 2001.

7. *Constraints to scaling up the health Millennium Development Goals: costing and financial gap analysis.* Geneva, World Health Organization, 2010 (Background document for the Taskforce on Innovative International Financing for Health Systems; http://www.internationalhealthpartnership.net//CMS_files/documents/working_group_1_technical_background_report_(world_health_organization)_EN.pdf, accessed 6 July 2010).

8. Durairaj V. *Fiscal space for health in resource-poor countries.* World health report 2010 background paper, no. 41 (http://www.who.int/healthsystems/topics/financing/healthreport/whr_background/en).

9. Missoni E, Solimano G. *Towards universal health coverage: the Chilean experience.* World health report 2010 background paper, no. 4 (http://www.who.int/healthsystems/topics/financing/healthreport/whr_background/en).

10. *Technical briefing on Millennium Development Goals.* Geneva, World Health Organization, 2010 (http://www.who.int/entity/gho/mdg/MDG_WHA2010.pdf, accessed 7 July 2010).

11. *World health statistics 2010.* Geneva, World Health Organization, 2010.

12. African Summit on HIV/AIDS, tuberculosis and other related infectious diseases. *Abuja Declaration on HIV/AIDS, Tuberculosis and Other Related Infectious Diseases, 24–27 April 2001.* Organisation of African Unity, 2001 (OAU/SPS/ABUJA/3).

13. Wibulpolprasert S, Thaiprayoon S. Thailand: good practice in expanding health care coverage. Lessons from reforms in a country in transition. In: Gottret P, Schieber GJ, Waters HR, eds. *Lessons from reforms in low- and middle-income countries. Good practices in health financing.* Washington, DC, The World Bank, 2008:355–384.

14. James CD, Dodd R, Nguyen K. *External aid and health spending in Viet Nam: additional or fungible?* World health report 2010 background paper, no. 40 (http://www.who.int/healthsystems/topics/financing/healthreport/whr_background/en).

15. Fernandes Antunes AF et al. *General budget support – has it benefited the health sector?* World health report 2010 background paper, no. 14 (http://www.who.int/healthsystems/topics/financing/healthreport/whr_background/en).

16. Kaddar M, Furrer E. Are current debt relief initiatives an option for scaling up health financing in beneficiary countries? *Bulletin of the World Health Organization,* 2008,86:877-883. doi:10.2471/BLT.08.053686 PMID:19030694

17. Gordon R, Li W. Tax structures in developing countries: many puzzles and a possible explanation. *Journal of Public Economics,* 2009,93:855-866. doi:10.1016/j.jpubeco.2009.04.001

18. Brondolo J et al. *Tax administration reform and fiscal adjustment: the case of Indonesia (2001–07).* Washington, DC, International Monetary Fund, 2008 (IMF Working Paper WP/08/129; http://www.imf.org/external/pubs/ft/wp/2008/wp08129.pdf, accessed 09 July, 2010).

19. *Promoting transparency and exchange of information for tax purposes.* Paris, Organisation for Economic Co-operation and Development, 2010 (http://www.oecd.org/dataoecd/32/45/43757434.pdf, accessed 7 July 2010).

20. Cummings RG et al. Tax morale affects tax compliance: evidence from surveys and an artefactual field experiment. *Journal of Economic Behavior & Organization,* 2009,70:447-457. doi:10.1016/j.jebo.2008.02.010

21.. Tsounta E. *Universal health care 101: lessons for the Eastern Caribbean and beyond.* Washington, DC, International Monetary Fund, 2009 (IMF Working Paper WP/09/61; http://www.imf.org/external/pubs/ft/wp/2009/wp0961.pdf, accessed 5 July 2010).

22. Witter S, Garshong B. Something old or something new? Social health insurance in Ghana. *BMC International Health and Human Rights*, 2009,9:20- doi:10.1186/1472-698X-9-20 PMID:19715583

23. Wanert S. *Aspects organisationnels du système de financement de la santé Français avec une attention générale pour la Réforme de l'Assurance Maladie Obligatoire du 13 août 2004.* Geneva, World Health Organization, 2009 (Health Systems Financing Discussion Paper No. 5, HSS/HSF/DP.F.09.5; http://www.who.int/health_financing/documents/cov-dp_f_09_05-org_fra-e/en/index.html, accessed 6 July 2010).

24. Unitaid, 2010 (http://www.unitaid.eu/en/UNITAID-Mission.html, accessed 1 June 2010).

25. Fryatt R, Mills A, Nordstrom A. Financing of health systems to achieve the health Millennium Development Goals in low-income countries. *Lancet*, 2010,375:419-426. doi:10.1016/S0140-6736(09)61833-X PMID:20113826

26. *Questions and answers.* Unitaid (http://www.unitaid.eu/images/NewWeb/documents/en_qa_finalrevised_mar10.pdf, accessed 7 July 2010).

27. Le Gargasson J-B, Salomé B. *The role of innovative financing mechanisms for health.* World health report 2010 background paper, no.12 (http://www.who.int/healthsystems/topics/financing/healthreport/whr_background/en).

28. *MassiveGood.* Millenium Foundation (http://www.massivegood.org/en_US/the-project, accessed 7 July 2010).

29. International Financing Facility for Immunization (IFFIm) (http://www.iff-immunisation.org, accessed 3 May 2010).

30. *Raising and channeling funds: Working Group 2 report.* Taskforce on Innovative International Financing for Health Systems, 2009 (http://www.internationalhealthpartnership.net//CMS_files/documents/working_group_2_report:_raising_and_channeling_funds_EN.pdf, accessed 6 July 2010).

31. *Currency transaction levy.* Taskforce on Innovative International Financing for Health Systems (http://www.internationalhealthpartnership.net//CMS_files/documents/factsheet_-_currency_transaction_levy_EN.pdf, accessed 6 June 2010).

32. Honohan P, Yoder S. *Financial transactions tax panacea, threat, or damp squib?* Washington, DC, The World Bank, 2010 (Policy Research Working Paper No. 5230; http://www-wds.worldbank.org/external/default/WDSContentServer/IW3P/IB/2010/03/02/000158349_20100302153508/Rendered/PDF/WPS5230.pdf, accessed 7 July 2007).

33. *Mobile phone voluntary solidarity contribution (VSC).* Taskforce on Innovative International Financing for Health Systems Factsheet, 2010 (http://www.internationalhealthpartnership.net//CMS_files/documents/factsheet_-_mobile_phone_voluntary_solidarity_contribution_EN.pdf, accessed 30 May 2010).

34. Holt E. Romania mulls over fast food tax. *Lancet*, 2010,375:1070- doi:10.1016/S0140-6736(10)60462-X PMID:20352658

35. Bank for International Settlements. *Triennial Central Bank Survey: foreign exchange and derivatives market activity in 2007.* Basel, Bank for International Settlements, 2007 (http://www.bis.org/publ/rpfxf07t.pdf, accessed 12 July 2010).

36. Musango L, Aboubacar I. *Assurance maladie obligatoire au Gabon: un atout pour le bien-être de la population.* World health report 2010 background paper, no. 16 (http://www.who.int/healthsystems/topics/financing/healthreport/whr_background/en).

37. Stenberg K et al. *Responding to the challenge of resource mobilization - mechanisms for raising additional domestic resources for health.* World health report 2010 background paper, no. 13 (http://www.who.int/healthsystems/topics/financing/healthreport/whr_background/en).

38. NishtarS Choked pipes–reforming Pakistan's mixed health system. Oxford, Oxford University Press, 2010

39. Prakongsai P, Patcharanarumol W, Tangcharoensathien V. Can earmarking mobilize and sustain resources to the health sector? *Bulletin of the World Health Organization*, 2008,86:898-901. doi:10.2471/BLT.07.049593 PMID:19030701

40. Bayarsaikhan D, Muiser J. *Financing health promotion.* Geneva, World Health Organization, 2007 (Health Systems Financing Discussion Paper No. 4, HSS/HSF/DP.07.4; http://www.who.int/health_financing/documents/dp_e_07_4-health_promotion.pdf, accessed 6 July 2010).

41. Srithamrongswat S et al. *Funding health promotion and prevention – the Thai experience.* World health report 2010 background paper, no. 48 (http://www.who.int/healthsystems/topics/financing/healthreport/whr_background/en) .

42. Tangcharoensathien V et al. Innovative financing of health promotion. In: Heggenhougen K, Quah S, eds. *International Encyclopedia of Public Health*, 1st edn. San Diego, CA, Academic Press, 2008:624–637.

43. Doetinchem O. *Hypothecation of tax revenue for health.* World health report 2010 background paper, no. 51 (http://www.who.int/healthsystems/topics/financing/healthreport/whr_background/en).

44. Nemtsov AV. Alcohol-related harm and alcohol consumption in Moscow before, during and after a major anti-alcohol campaign. *Addiction*, 1998,93:1501-1510. PMID:9926554

45. Ravishankar N et al. Financing of global health: tracking development assistance for health from 1990 to 2007. *Lancet*, 2009,373:2113-2124. doi:10.1016/S0140-6736(09)60881-3 PMID:19541038

46. *Development aid rose in 2009 and most donors will meet 2010 aid targets.* Paris, Organisation for Economic Co-operation and Development, 2010 (http://www.oecd.org/document/11/0,3343,en_2649_34487_44981579_1_1_1_1,00.html, accessed 7 June 2010).

47. Piva P, Dodd R. Where did all the aid go? An in-depth analysis of increased health aid flows over the past 10 years. *Bulletin of the World Health Organization*, 2009,87:930-939. doi:10.2471/BLT.08.058677 PMID:20454484

48. Goldsborough D. *Does the IMF constrain health spending in poor countries? Evidence and an agenda for action.* Washington, DC, Center for Global Development, 2007 (http://www.cgdev.org/doc/IMF/IMF_Report.pdf, accessed 3 May 2007).

49. *Changing IMF policies to get more doctors, nurses and teachers hired in developing countries.* ActionAid, 2010 (http://www.ifiwatchnet.org/sites/ifiwatchnet.org/files/4-pager%20--%20IMF%20and%20health.pdf, accessed 7 July 2010).

50. Rowden R. *Viewpoint: restrictive IMF policies undermine efforts at health systems strengthening.* World health report 2010 background paper, no. 49 (http://www.who.int/healthsystems/topics/financing/healthreport/whr_backgroundbackground/en) .

51. *The IMF and aid to Sub-Saharan Africa.* Washington, DC, Independent Evaluation Office of the International Monetary Fund, 2007 (http://www.imf.org/external/np/ieo/2007/ssa/eng/pdf/report.pdf, accessed 7 July 2010).

52. Sanjeev G, Powell R, Yang Y. *Macroeconomic challenges of scaling up aid to Africa: a checklist for practitioners.* Washington, DC, International Monetary Fund, 2006 (http://www.imf.org/external/pubs/ft/afr/aid/2006/eng/aid.pdf, accessed 12 July 2010).

53. Haacker M. *Macroeconomic constraints to health financing: a guide for the perplexed.* World health report 2010 background paper, no. 50 (http://www.who.int/healthsystems/topics/financing/healthreport/whr_background/en).

54. Gostin LO et al. *The joint learning initiative on national and global responsibility for health.* World health report 2010 background paper, no. 53 (http://www.who.int/healthsystems/topics/financing/healthreport/whr_background/en).

55. Ooms G, Derderian K, Melody D. Do we need a world health insurance to realise the right to health? *PLoS Medicine*, 2006,3:e530- doi:10.1371/journal.pmed.0030530 PMID:17194201

56. Development Assistance [online database]. Paris, Organisation for Economic Co-operation and Development (OECD) (http://www.oecd.org/dac/stats/idsonline, accessed 3 March 2010).

57. *The world health report 2006: working together for health.* Geneva, World Health Organization, 2006.

58. *Effective aid – better health: report prepared for the Accra High–level Forum on Aid Effectiveness.* The World Bank/Organisation for Economic Co-operation and Development/World Health Organization, 2008 (http://www.gavialliance.org/resources/effectiveaid_betterhealth_en.pdf, accessed 28 February 2010).

59. *The Paris Declaration on Aid Effectiveness and the Accra Agenda for Action.* Paris, Organisation for Economic Co-operation and Development, 2008 (http://www.oecd.org/dataoecd/11/41/34428351.pdf, accessed 7 July 2010).

60. *Working Group 2: Raising and channelling funds – progress report to taskforce.* Taskforce on Innovative International Financing for Health Systems, 2009 (http://www.internationalhealthpartnership.net/pdf/IHP%20Update%2013/Taskforce/london%20meeting/new/Working%20Group%202%20First%20Report%20090311.pdf, accessed 19 May 2010).

61. Waddington C et al. *Global aid architecture and the health Millennium Development Goals.* Norwegian Agency for Development Cooperation, 2009 (www.norad.no/en/_attachment/146678/binary/79485?download=true, accessed 5 April 2010).

62. Van de Maele N. *Variability in disbursements of aid for health by donor and recipient.* World health report 2010 background paper, no. 15 (http://www.who.int/healthsystems/topics/financing/healthreport/whr_background/en).

End notes

a   The high-level taskforce included interventions proven to reduce mortality among mothers, newborns and children under five; childbirth care; reproductive health services; prevention and treatment of the main infectious diseases; diagnosis, information, referral, and palliative care for any presenting conditions; and health promotion.

b   Typically, the term official development assistance (ODA) is used to describe assistance provided officially by governments. Development assistance for health is broader, including ODA, plus lending and credits from multilateral development banks, transfers from major foundations and NGOs.

Chapter 3 | Strength in numbers

Key messages

- Systems requiring direct payments at the time people need care – including user fees and payments for medicines – prevent millions from accessing services and result in financial hardship, even impoverishment, for millions more.

- Countries can accelerate progress towards universal coverage by reducing reliance on direct payments. This requires introducing or strengthening forms of prepayment and pooling.

- The countries that have come closest to ensuring universal health coverage mandate contributions for people who can afford to pay, through taxation and/or insurance contributions.

- Compulsory prepaid funds should ideally be combined in one pool rather than be kept in separate funds. By reducing fragmentation, there is an increased potential to provide financial protection from a given level of prepaid funds, which in turn makes it easier to achieve equity goals.

- Voluntary schemes, such as community health insurance or microinsurance, can still play a useful role where compulsory sources provide only minimal levels of prepayment. If they are able to redirect some of their direct payments into prepaid pools, they can expand protection to some extent against the financial risks of ill health and help people understand the benefits of being insured.

- Some people will face financial barriers to access even if direct payments are eliminated; transport and accommodation costs to obtain treatment might still prove prohibitive. Governments must consider options, including conditional cash transfers, for reducing these barriers.

3

Strength in numbers

The problems with direct payments

How health services are paid for is a key aspect of health system performance. While raising sufficient resources is obviously imperative to running a health system, how those resources are used to buy goods and services – how payment is effected, in other words – is just as important. One of the most common forms of payment around the globe is direct payment for medicines and health services at the time of need, and it is the poorer countries that rely on it most (*1*).

A recent study of 50 low- and middle-income countries based on WHO health wexpenditure data, a health systems typology survey and interviews with key informants, revealed that only six of the countries did not require direct payment of some form at government facilities (*3*).

But direct payment is not restricted to lower-income countries or less-sophisticated health financing systems (Fig. 3.1). Charging users when they request care is the predominant fund-raising mechanism in 33 countries and accounts for more than 25% of all the funds raised for health in another 75 (*4*). As we saw in Chapter 1, direct payments take many forms, including doctor consultation fees, payments for procedures, medicines and other supplies, and for laboratory tests. They can also come in the form of deductibles, such as co-insurance and co-payments for people covered by insurance.

One of the reasons direct payment is unsuited to the delivery/consumption of health care is that it inhibits access. This is especially true for poorer people, who must often choose between paying for health and paying for other necessities such as food or rent. For people who feel they simply must receive treatment – for the growing lump in the breast or the child's fever that will not come down – there is the risk of impoverishment or even destitution. Burundi introduced user fees in 2002. Two years later, four out of five patients were either in debt or had sold assets (*5*). In many countries, people are forced to borrow or sell assets to finance health care (*6, 7*).

The incidence of financial catastrophe associated with direct payments for health services – i.e. the proportion of people who spend out of pocket more than 40% of their incomes after deducting expenses for food each year – can be as high as 11% per year at a national level and is typically more than 2% in low-income countries. Perhaps not surprisingly, within countries the incidence is generally lowest among

> *"User fees have punished the poor."*
>
> Dr Margaret Chan (2)

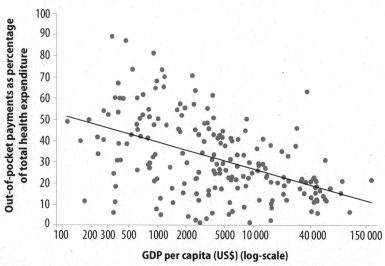

Fig. 3.1. **Out-of-pocket payments as a function of gross domestic product (GDP) per capita, 2007**

Source (4).

richer people, but the poorest do not always suffer most in this specific financial sense because they cannot afford to use services at all and do not incur health expenses. Recent research also suggests that households with a disabled member and those with children or elderly members are more likely to experience catastrophic health expenditures (8–11).

It is only when the reliance on direct payments falls to less than 15–20% of total health expenditures that the incidence of financial catastrophe routinely falls to negligible levels (Fig. 3.2) (1). It is largely the high-income countries that have achieved these levels, so low- and middle-income countries might wish to set themselves more attainable short-term goals. The countries of the South-East Asia and Western Pacific Regions of WHO, for example, recently set themselves a target of 30–40% (12, 13).

Even when relatively low, any kind of charge imposed directly on households may discourage using health-care services or push people living close to poverty under the poverty line. An experimental study in Kenya showed that introducing a US$ 0.75 fee for previously free insecticide-treated bed nets decreased demand by 75% (14), while the introduction of a small charge for de-worming drugs reduced uptake by 80% (15). Direct payments, however small, may also encourage inappropriate self-treatment and self-medication – the use of dated or substandard medicines or partial doses, for example – or postponing often crucial early consultations with a health professional (16).

Direct payments do not have to be official to restrict access. In Armenia, for example, until recently only about 10% of direct payments at hospitals were official user charges levied by government facilities. A substantial portion of the other 90% was made up of the unofficial or informal payments to health workers. The government has now devised strategies to eliminate unofficial payments, recognizing that they, too, prevent people from accessing needed care and introduce an added layer of anxiety for the sick and their families because of the unpredictable nature of unofficial rates (17). Informal payments are found in many countries all around the world (18–20).

Direct payments are the least equitable form of health funding. They are regressive, allowing the rich to pay the same amount as the poor for any particular service. Socioeconomic background is not the only basis for inequality. In cultures where women have a lower status than men, women and girls must often wait for treatment behind the men of the household when user fees are charged, and therefore, are less likely to access services (21).

The benefit derived from direct payments is restricted to the individual served and the provider or facility that collects the fee. A coin given to a nurse in a village clinic ensures the paying individual obtains a service or medicines. This is not bad in itself, but it is bad if, as health minister, you want to help also the people in the surrounding hills who may not have any coins to offer. Direct payments tend to preclude spreading the cost across groups of people in formalized expressions of solidarity – between the rich and poor, for example, or between the healthy and the sick. They also make it impossible to spread costs over an individual's lifetime. With direct payment, people cannot pay contributions when they are young and healthy, then draw on them as needed later in life. They must pay when they are sick. They must pay when they are most vulnerable.

Fig. 3.2. **The effect of out-of-pocket spending on financial catastrophe and impoverishment**

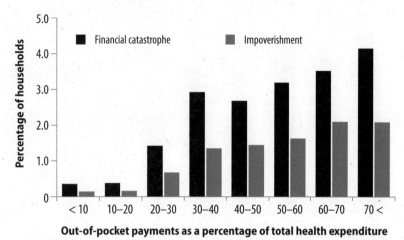

Out-of-pocket payments as a percentage of total health expenditure

Source (1).

Given the shortcomings of direct payment as a health financing mechanism, why is it so widespread?

First, a high reliance on direct payments is found when governments are unwilling to spend more on health or do not believe or understand that they have the capacity to expand prepayment and pooling systems. This leaves a gap between necessary service coverage and the coverage the government does manage to provide. Typically, health workers are caught in the middle, making do with low salaries (supplemented sometimes with informal charges) while trying to provide services with limited supplies and medicines. In these scenarios, many governments have chosen to implement formal user fees or co-payments to supplement health worker salaries and make medicines and supplies more available.

Second, direct payments offer the opportunity to tap into resources in areas where health facilities might otherwise have no money at all – perhaps in areas where government funding arrives irregularly, if at all. In the Democratic Republic of the Congo, geographical remoteness, sporadic conflict and natural disasters have sometimes isolated, at least temporarily, many parts of the country. This isolation from government support and control, especially in the eastern provinces, made direct payment from patients the default method (aside from external aid) to keep the services running, at least at some level (22). Direct payments commonly become the default method of financing health in the aftermath of crises, notably after a period of armed conflict. At a time when people most need access to health services, many simply cannot afford to be treated (23).

Third, direct payment can seem like an attractive option during periods of economic recession. In fact, the first wave of user fees for health services at government facilities in developing countries was catalysed by the 1970s global recession. The global debt crisis sparked the structural adjustment policies that restricted government spending (24). At that time it was suggested that charging fees might be a way to generate the needed additional revenue, reduce overuse and encourage the provision of services that carried low charges and costs (25).

The 1987 Bamako Initiative was one of the outcomes of that type of thinking. Approved by African health ministers, the initiative built on a rationale that, in the context of a chronically underresourced public health sector, direct payments would ensure at least some funding to pay for needed medicines and, sometimes, staff at the local level (26). There is evidence that reforms inspired by Bamako improved the availability of services and medicines in some contexts, but there is other evidence that direct payments also created barriers to access, especially for the poor (27–31).

Finally, many countries impose some form of direct payment, often to curb the overuse of health services, as a form of cost-containment. This is a relatively blunt instrument for controlling costs and has the unwanted side-effect of deterring use in some of the population groups who need it most. It will be discussed further in Chapter 4.

Do exemptions from charges work?

Most countries that rely on direct payments try to avoid the exclusion they give rise to by exempting specific groups – pregnant women or children, for example – or by providing certain procedures free of charge. In 2006, the Burundi government waived fees on maternal and child care, including deliveries. Three months after this fee exemption was implemented, the use of outpatient services for children under five increased by 42% (32). Senegal removed user fees for deliveries and caesarean sections in 2005; according to the first round of evaluations, this policy lead to a 10% increase in deliveries in public health facilities and more than a 30% increase in caesarean sections (33).

Income has also been used to assess eligibility for exemptions. Germany, for example, imposes co-payments for some services, but only up to a limit determined by the person's income. France also offers free complementary insurance – insurance to cover co-payments – to the poor (34). But exemption schemes based on income have been shown to be less efficient in lower-income countries. Where most people are subsistence farmers or not in formal wage employment, it is difficult for means-testers to identify which people are the poorest. They are caught between using broad categories to avoid excluding deserving groups – an approach that leads to benefits going to the less deserving – and too-strict criteria that give rise to undercoverage, leaving the barriers to access more or less in place (35).

Simply declaring exemptions is unlikely to be sufficient in most settings. In Cambodia, for example, an assessment of the impact of user fees five years after their introduction in the 1990s showed that exemptions were ineffective: because 50% of the fee income was redistributed to health staff, each exemption case represented a loss of income for poorly paid health workers (36). To be effective, exemptions require a funding mechanism to compensate facilities for potential lost revenues. Cambodia subsequently took such a course. Health equity funds were introduced, with funding from specific donor agencies, to compensate health facilities and staff for lost revenues when granting exemptions to the poor.

This was associated with an increased use of health facilities by the poorest groups, in both urban and rural settings (37, 38). There have also been gains in financial risk protection; borrowing money to pay for care was lower for health equity funds' beneficiaries than for fee-paying patients (39). Support for this approach has grown, with the health equity funds now being financed mostly through the pooled donor funds in the Cambodian Health Sector Support Project, although since 2007, they have also attracted more domestic funds from the ministry of economy and finance. A similar approach was taken in Kyrgyzstan (40).

But there are other factors that deter poor people from using services even when exemptions or subsidies to cover their costs are available, factors that are more difficult to quantify: poor people's reluctance to be stigmatized by seeking an exemption or a subsidy, for example, or the way health workers sometimes treat the poor. Where health workers are dependent or partially dependent on direct payments for their income, there is a clear incentive to refuse requests for exemption. A World Bank study found that facilities in Kenya rarely granted more than two waivers per month to the entire population, 42% of which lived below the poverty line (41). As troubling as that might be, we should bear in mind that health workers often struggle on inadequate salaries.

On the other hand, it appears that targeting by income might work in some settings, especially at the community level. In Cambodia, for example, community leaders were asked to determine who should be exempted from fees to be financed by the health equity fund. Their assessment proved accurate, at least to the extent that the people selected for exemptions were more destitute than those not selected (42). In Pakistan, the HeartFile project is exploring innovative exemption mechanisms that will be evaluated shortly (43).

Several countries that were part of the former Soviet Union found the levels of public spending on health declining rapidly in the 1990s, with a subsequent rapid growth in informal out-of-pocket payments. This created severe financial barriers to care for those unable to pay. As a result, many of these countries introduced formal fees or co-payments designed to curtail informal payments and raise additional resources. They then had to introduce exemption mechanisms to identify and protect those unable to pay (44). Despite this, many of these countries still have relatively high rates of financial catastrophe linked to direct payments for health services (45).

The retreat from direct payments

The practical problems that hamper efforts to target specific groups dissolve when policy-makers expand exemptions to the entire population. Six low-income countries have recently abolished direct payments in government facilities, and one extended the policy to nongovernmental organization health facilities (46). In some cases, this action significantly increases the number of people seeking treatment. Removing fees in rural Zambia in April 2006 and January 2007, for example, resulted in a 55% increase in the use of government facilities; districts with a greater concentration of poor people recorded the biggest increases (47). Attendance rates at health centres in Uganda jumped 84% when fees were scrapped in 2001 (48).

However, in both these cases, abolishing fees was not a stand-alone measure; increasing rural health facility budgets was an integral part of the policy. In Zambia, increased allocations from domestic sources, combined with donor support, meant the districts received 36% more in budget support than they had received from user fees in the previous year. The Ugandan government increased spending for medicines and gave facility managers more control over budget funds so that they would not lose the flexibility previously derived from fees.

Some observers have argued that direct charges at government facilities can be eliminated without too much pain because they have generated only limited income (49, 50). Studies on official user fees at government facilities in 16 sub-Saharan countries revealed they generated on average 5% of total recurrent health system expenditure, not including administrative costs (51, 52).

However, budgeted funds are largely tied up with the fixed costs of staff and infrastructure, leaving little for key patient treatment inputs, such as medicines and other disposable items. This is where revenues from fees often play a critical role. A study from one region of Ghana revealed that while direct payments provided only 8% and 27% of the total expenditures of a sample of health centres and hospitals, respectively, they accounted for 66% (health centres) and 83% (hospitals) of non-salary expenditures, constituting an important part of the only relatively flexible funds under the facility managers' control (53).

Whatever their precise value within a system, policy-makers must consider the consequences of removing direct payments. Without context-specific planning for increased demand and lost fees, abolishing them can result in under- or unpaid and overworked staff, empty medicine dispensaries and poorly maintained or broken equipment (46, 54). It is worth noting that the incidence of catastrophic health expenditure among the poor did not fall after the abolition of user fees in Uganda, most likely because the frequent unavailability of drugs at government facilities after 2001 forced some patients to go to private pharmacies (55). It is also possible that informal payments to health workers increased to offset the lost user-fee revenue.

A return to informal payment appears to be one of the attendant risks of withdrawing user fees, although the extent to which this happens is not clear. Nor is it clear whether the countries that introduced official fees to try to curtail informal payments have managed to eliminate them despite some success in reducing them (56).

These experiences show that to reduce dependence on direct payment – a major obstacle to universal coverage – it is essential to find resources elsewhere to replace the official or unofficial money that was formerly paid. This can occur directly if governments are able and willing to channel more funds into health (57). But there are alternatives to simply spending more that involve making other changes to the financing system.

Such alternatives are not only for the most resource-constrained countries to consider. Although direct payments play a relatively unimportant

role in most countries of the Organisation for Economic Co-operation and Development (OECD), an upward trend in direct payments was evidenced in many even before the global economic downturn. Many had increased patient cost sharing through direct payments to limit government contributions and discourage the unnecessary use of services (58). These direct payments create financial hardship for some people and reduce access to services for others. As we noted in Chapter 1, direct payments result in more than 1% of the population, or almost four million of people, suffering catastrophic payments each year in just six OECD countries.

Strength in numbers

The most effective way to deal with the financial risk of paying for health services is to share it, and the more people who share, the better the protection. Had Narin Pintalakarn joined with the people in his village to set up an emergency fund to be drawn on in cases of illness or accident, the cost of his brain surgery and care at Khon Kaen Regional Hospital would have exhausted its reserves. Fortunately, he banded together with Thailand's tax-paying public, which finances the universal coverage scheme. This was not a conscious decision; it was a decision taken and fought for by others over many decades. Pintalakarn was part of such a large group of people that even though, as a casual labourer earning the equivalent of US$ 5 a day, he was unable to contribute a single baht at the time of his care, he could still be treated and made well again. There is strength in numbers (Box 3.1).

People have long been voluntarily pooling their money to protect themselves against the financial risk of paying for health services. The Students' Health Home insurance scheme started in West Bengal in 1952 and schemes in several western African countries, including Benin, Guinea, Mali, Senegal, have been operating since the 1980s, often with no more

Box 3.1. **Strength in numbers**

Policy-makers planning to move away from user fees and other forms of direct payments have three interrelated options. The first is to replace direct payments with forms of prepayment, most commonly a combination of taxes and insurance contributions. The second is to consolidate existing pooled funds into larger pools, and the third is to improve the efficiency with which funds are used (this is the topic of Chapter 4).

Prepayment does not necessarily mean that people pay the full costs of the care they will receive, but that they make payments in advance. It means they contribute to a pool that they, or others, can draw on in the event of illness. In some years, they may receive services that cost more than their contributions, and in some years, less.

Whether or not pools are consolidated into one national pool, or kept separate to stimulate competition or to reflect the needs of different regions, is partly a matter of national preference. In most high-income countries, collecting and pooling happens at the level of central government – with the collecting and pooling functions split between the ministry of finance, or the treasury, and the ministry of health. The Republic of Korea, for example, chose to merge more than 300 individual insurers into a single national fund (59).

But there are exceptions. Swiss citizens have voted overwhelmingly to keep multiple pools rather than go for a single *caisse unique* and resources are pooled for smaller groups of people (60). The Netherlands has had a system of competing funds since the early 1990s (61). In both cases, insurance contributions are compulsory and both governments seek to consolidate the pools, at least to some extent, through risk equalization, whereby money is transferred from insurance funds that service a greater proportion of low-risk people to those that insure predominantly high-risk people and thereby incur higher costs.

Nevertheless, experience suggests that a single pool offers several advantages, including greater efficiency (see Chapter 4) and capacity for cross-subsidization within the population. There is strong evidence that fragmented pooling systems without risk equalization can work against equity goals in financing, because each pool has an incentive to enrol low-risk people and the parts of the population that receive more benefits are unwilling to share their pooled funds with the parts of the population that are worse off (62).

Risk equalization also takes place when central governments allocate funds for health to lower levels of government or to health facilities in different geographical areas. The people and businesses in richer regions with fewer health problems generally contribute more to the pool in taxes and charges than they receive, while those living in poorer regions with greater health problems receive more than they contribute. Some countries also use complex allocation formulae to decide what are fair allocations to the various geographical areas and facilities (63).

than a few hundred members (64–67). These schemes are highly localized, often tied to a village or a group of professionals. In Ukraine, for example, individuals have formed so-called sickness funds to help meet the costs of medicines where there is limited budgetary provision to local health facilities. Contributions are usually about 5% of wages and often supplemented by money raised at charitable events. While coverage is small when measured at the national level, the funds play an important role in some small towns with underfunded health facilities (68).

In the absence of an effective alternative – a functioning publicly regulated pooling mechanism – such schemes often prove popular among different population groups. A total of 49 health-related community schemes operate in Bangladesh, India and Nepal, with the Indian schemes serving informal workers such as labourers and small farmers. These schemes can have hundreds of thousands of members (69), but in relative terms, they are generally too small to function effectively as risk pools, providing only limited coverage for expensive interventions such as surgery. They do, however, offer a degree of protection, covering primary-level care costs, and in some cases, part of the cost of hospitalization; they also familiarize people with prepayment and pooling, and can engender the solidarity needed to build a wider movement towards universal coverage (70).

Community health insurance, or microinsurance, can also be an institutional stepping stone to bigger regional schemes, which in turn, can be consolidated into national risk pools, although this almost always requires government encouragement. Many of the countries that have moved closest to universal coverage started with smaller voluntary health insurance schemes that gradually consolidated into compulsory social insurance for specific groups, finally achieving much higher levels of financial risk protection in much larger pools. Voluntary health insurance schemes were important in helping to develop, many years later, universal coverage in Germany and Japan.

More recently, several countries have chosen a more direct route to universal coverage than was followed by Germany and Japan a century ago. Prior to the universal coverage reforms that began in 2001, Thailand ran several separate schemes: the Health Welfare Scheme for the Poor, the Voluntary Health Card scheme, the Civil Servants Medical Benefit Scheme, the Social Security Scheme for the formal sector, and private insurance. Despite rapidly expanding coverage during the 1990s, about 30% of the Thai population was still without coverage in 2001 (71). The civil servants scheme also received a much greater government subsidy per member than did the Health Welfare Scheme for the Poor (72). In effect, these arrangements increased inequalities.

The universal coverage reform programme of 2001 moved rapidly to reduce the fragmented array of schemes and supply-side subsidies the government made to health facilities. Policy-makers rejected slowly expanding coverage through insurance contributions, recognizing that a large proportion of the people who remained uncovered were in informal employment and many were too poor to contribute insurance payments (73). Instead, they replaced the former Health Welfare and Voluntary Health

Card schemes, and used general budget revenues that previously flowed to these and to public providers, to create a national pool for what is now called the universal coverage scheme (previously the so-called 30 Baht scheme). The civil servants and the social security schemes remained separate, but the universal coverage scheme still pools funds for nearly 50 million people, and has reduced the proportion of the population without insurance coverage from 30% to less than 4%.

All countries using competing insurers for mandatory coverage use some system of risk equalization to avoid the negative effects of fragmentation. The Czech Republic started with a range of health insurers, but one fund shouldered the burden of a considerably older and poorer client base. In 2003 the government extended its risk equalization mechanism to all compulsory prepaid revenues for health insurance, effectively transferring resources from funds covering low-risk people to those covering higher-risk people. This reform also created a mechanism to compensate insurers for high-cost cases (74).

Where and how to cover more people?

In moving towards health financing based on prepayment and pooling, policy-makers must first decide which sections of the population are to be covered. Historically, many of the high-income countries in Europe and also Japan have begun with formal-sector workers, who are easy to identify and whose regular wage income is relatively easy to tax.

However, starting with the formal sector today would risk further fragmentation and inequality rather than move the system towards a large risk pool that enables subsidies to flow from rich to poor, and healthy to sick. Since 1980, perhaps only the Republic of Korea has moved towards universal coverage in this way. In that country, the system evolved under strong government leadership and amid rapid economic growth and high levels (compared with most low- and middle-income countries) of formal-worker participation (75, 76).

Elsewhere, results have been less positive. Typically, groups that initially receive coverage push for increased benefits or reduced contributions, but not to extend coverage to others, especially those unable to contribute. This exacerbates inequalities given that those in formal employment are generally more secure financially than the rest of the population. This was Mexico's experience 15 years ago when different types of pooled funds covered different population groups, each with different levels of benefits (77–79). Such arrangements are not only inequitable, but inefficient and costly (80, 81). This was the rationale for the more recent reforms in Mexico aiming to provide more effective coverage to the poorest groups (82).

Focusing on the poor

When planning to finance universal coverage, policy-makers must not exclude those who cannot contribute, perhaps because they do not earn enough to pay income taxes or make insurance contributions. The key issue is whether entitlements should be linked to contributions. Should those who do not contribute financially get free health care? What little research there is on this subject suggests that while most people believe the poor should get help with health-care costs, they also believe such help should stop short of paying for everything (*83*). Each country will see this issue through its own socioeconomic lens, but policy-makers must remember that health financing systems that are perceived to be fair have the best chance at long-term sustainability.

The danger of exclusion is not limited to the sick and the poor. There are the poor in dangerous jobs, for example. In the region where Narin Pintalakarn had his accident, labourers are the people most likely to end up in an intensive care unit or, if no provision has been made to pay for their treatment, in the village morgue.

Whatever system is adopted, some general government revenues will be needed to ensure that the people who cannot afford to contribute can still access health services, by subsidizing their health insurance premiums or by not imposing direct payments, for example. Where the combined total of expenditure from general government revenues and compulsory health insurance contributions is lower than about 5–6% of gross domestic product (GDP), countries struggle to ensure health service coverage for the poor (*84*). The WHO Regional Office for the Americas advocates for a 6% level (*85, 86*). Only the richer countries achieve this level of compulsory pooling, but countries aiming for universal coverage need to develop strategies for expanding contributions that will cover the poor over time. This can be done in many ways, including subsidizing insurance contributions or providing services at no charge.

While who is to be covered needs careful consideration, where the money comes from – whether from general government revenues, or some form of compulsory health insurance contribution – is less of an issue. In fact, breaking down the options into a tax/social health insurance dichotomy can be unhelpful. In most health financing systems, hybridization prevails, the collection, pooling and expenditure of resources relying on a mix of mechanisms. Sources of revenue do not necessarily determine how funds are pooled or who benefits. Insurance contributions made by employers and/or employees can be put into the same pool as contributions from general government revenues. In the Republic of Moldova, the government introduced its National Health Insurance Company in 2004, drawing on two main sources of funds: a new tax of 4% was levied on wages (increased to 7% in 2009); and general budget revenues that previously flowed to district and national health facilities were redirected to the company (*87*).

Pooling general budget revenues with compulsory insurance contributions virtually eliminated the fragmentation of the decentralized budgetary system and, when combined with a shift from input- to output-based payment methods, led to greater equalization in per capita government health spending across local government areas. There was also a decline in the level of out-of-pocket payment for the poorest 20% of the population (*88, 89*), though the Republic of Moldova still faces challenges in extending coverage to segments of its population (Box 3.2).

Even Germany, which is regarded as having the world's oldest employment-based social health insurance, has increased the share of general government revenues in the insurance pool. This move was a response to the challenges posed by an ageing population and the resulting dwindling base for wage-linked health insurance contributions. The country has also had to consider the impact of the global economic crisis that began in 2008 on employment and contribution rates. Subsequently, Germany has injected additional funds from general government revenues into the insurance system and reduced wage-based health insurance contribution rates from 15.5% to 14.9% (*91, 92*).

Other barriers to access

While moving from direct payments to a system of prepayment and pooling helps poorer people obtain care, it does not guarantee access. Direct payments are only one of the financial costs people face in seeking health services, and user fees paid at government facilities can be a small proportion of these costs. Furthermore, financial costs are only one of the potential barriers to care (*93, 94*). There are cultural and language barriers in societies that are multicultural, for example, where women are prevented from travelling by themselves in some settings.

Results from the World Health Surveys in 39 low- and lower-middle-income countries show than, on average, only 45% of the total out-of-pocket costs of outpatient care were for payments at government facilities, including doctors' fees, medicines and tests (the grey segments in Fig. 3.3). In some countries, it was less than 15%. The remaining 55% represented payments to private facilities, including nongovernmental organizations, and for medicines and tests bought privately (*95*). Offering health services that are free in government facilities only goes part of the way to lowering financial barriers to access; in some countries, it is quite a small part.

Transport can be another major expense, especially in remote rural areas. The same World Health Surveys study of 39 countries showed that transport costs represented, on average, more than 10% of total out-of-pocket payments incurred when people sought health care (*95*). Transport costs can also persuade people to delay treatment (*96*). A prolonged stay in hospital often necessitates accommodation and meals for carers. This, too, adds to the

---

Box 3.2. The Republic of Moldova entitlement issues

The Republic of Moldova introduced a national system of mandatory health insurance in 2004. Laws stipulate that the economically active population make contributions through a payroll tax, or if self-employed, pay a flat-rate contribution. The remainder of the population, including those registered as unemployed or non-working, is exempt from making contributions and insured by the government, which makes a contribution on their behalf. The shift in the basis of entitlement from being a citizen of the Republic of Moldova to being an individual who pays a premium has meant that about one quarter of the population (27.6% in 2009) has inadequate access to health care. These people, rural agricultural workers for the most part, do have access to life-saving services and a limited number of consultations with primary health care providers, but all other services must be paid for directly, out of pocket (*87*).

Not only did the government demand that these people – many living below the poverty line – pay a premium, that premium is fixed for all self-insured people, including doctors, notaries and lawyers. Another law was passed in February 2009, which ensures that all those registered as poor under the recently approved Law on Social Support will automatically receive fully subsidized health insurance. Coverage concerns were further addressed through legislation approved in December 2009 that expanded significantly (e.g. all primary care) the package of services for all citizens regardless of their insurance status. Despite some persisting equity issues, the centralizing of all public funding for health care and the split between purchasing and providing functions has led to greater geographical equity in government health spending per capita since the health insurance reform was introduced in 2004 (*90*).

cost of treatment (*97*). Even in settings where there are no or limited user fees, transport costs and other direct payments can be a significant impediment to households' receiving timely care (*98*).

There are several ways to overcome these additional financial barriers. One of the most obvious is to invest in primary care, ensuring everyone has inexpensive and easy physical access to services. This was a key factor in Thailand's movement towards universal coverage. Health financing reform was accompanied by a nationwide extension of primary care and a rural health service in which new medical school graduates were required to serve (*99*).

Other countries have opted for gradual reform, using vouchers or conditional cash transfers (CCTs) that give people the financial means to access services and/or undertake some specific health actions, usually linked to prevention (*100, 101*).

The use of these transfers has been most widespread in Latin America, where they have had some success in Brazil, Colombia, Honduras, Mexico and Nicaragua (*102–104*). In Mexico, the Oportunidades CCT scheme (previously known as Progresa), which started in 1997 and covers 5 million families with almost US$ 4 billion of public spending, has improved child health and reduced infant mortality (*105, 106*).

CCTs have also been implemented in a range of countries, including Bangladesh, Ecuador, Guatemala, India, Indonesia, Kenya, Nepal, Pakistan, Turkey and the USA. While they have their place in health financing, they are of little use in areas where services are limited or of poor quality, as is the case in much of rural sub-Saharan Africa.

CCTs and voucher schemes to offset the costs and lost income in seeking health care only work if they are targeted in a meaningful way. This means incurring potentially substantial costs and risking inefficiencies, such as leakage to the non-poor, who, because of their education or connections, are better able to exploit such benefits.

However, in areas where the barriers to access are substantial – poor, isolated rural areas, for instance – CCTs and voucher schemes may be the only short-term means to ensure people get the timely care they need.

Conclusion

The past three decades have provided lessons on the failings of direct payments such as user fees in financing health systems. The answer is to move towards a system of prepayment and pooling, sharing the financial risks of ill health across

Fig. 3.3. **Direct payments made at public and private facilities in 39 countries**

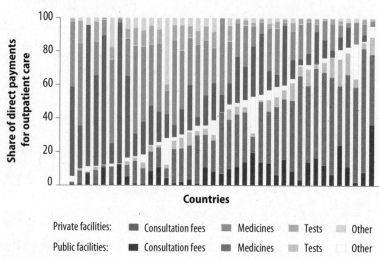

Source (*95*).

the largest population group possible. This must be carefully planned to avoid exacerbating the desperate situation of many of the world's poor and vulnerable, especially those living in remote areas. Box 3.3 summarizes the evidence presented in this chapter, information that can be used to inform country decision-making.

Long-term goals should be to lower the level of direct payments to below 15–20% of total health expenditure and to increase the proportion of combined government and compulsory insurance expenditure in GDP to about 5–6%. Reaching these targets will take time in some countries, which might set themselves more achievable short-term goals. The transition may seem daunting but great strides have recently been made by many countries, including countries with limited resources.

For those countries unable to generate the funding or lacking the technical capacity to support transition, external financial support will be vital. It is important that this support be given in the spirit of the Paris Declaration, in a way that allows aid recipients to formulate and execute their own national plans according to their priorities. The fragmented manner in which donors channel funds to countries should be avoided. Development partners also need to remember that many of the governments now relying on user fees introduced them in response to external advice and sometimes donors' requirements.

The transition to a system of prepayment and pooling requires action at the national and international level to honour lending commitments made over the past decade. Success will depend to a degree on the sustained mobilization of resources at the level to which governments have committed. Without investment in health services, especially in infrastructure and staff capable of delivering adequate primary-level care, the question of how health care is purchased is irrelevant. No care is no care, however you might want to pay for it.

Finally, even in countries where a system of prepayment and pooling is the norm, there will always be needy people for whom health care really must be free. ∎

Box 3.3. **Core ideas for reducing financial barriers**

The key question for today's decision-makers is this: how can we alter our existing health financing system to take advantage of the strength in numbers, or protect the gains that have been made? Here are some core considerations for policy-makers seeking to increase financial protection for the population while reducing barriers to using needed services.

Pooling pays

Countries can make faster progress towards universal coverage by introducing forms of prepayment and pooling to take advantage of the strength in numbers.

Consolidate or compensate

There are opportunities for improving coverage by consolidating fragmented pools, or by developing forms of risk compensation that enable the transfer of funds between them.

Combine tax and social health insurance

Where the funds come from does not have to determine how they are pooled. Taxes and insurance contributions can be combined to cover the population as a whole, rather than being kept in separate funds.

Compulsory contribution helps

Countries that have come closest to universal coverage use some form of compulsory contribution arrangement, whether they are funded by general government revenues or mandatory insurance contributions. This allows the pooled funds to cover the people who cannot pay found in all societies.

Voluntary schemes are a useful first step

Where the wider economic and fiscal context allows for only low levels of tax collection or compulsory insurance contributions, voluntary schemes have the potential to provide some protection against the financial risks of ill health and might help people understand the benefits of prepayment and pooling. But experience suggests that their potential is limited.

Drop direct payment

Only when household direct payments get to 15–20% of total health expenditures does the incidence of financial catastrophe decline to negligible levels, although countries and regions might wish to set themselves intermediate targets as we reported earlier for the South-East Asia and the Western Pacific Regions of WHO.

References

1. Xu K et al. *Exploring the thresholds of health expenditure for protection against financial risk.* World health report 2010 background paper, no. 19 (http://www.who.int/healthsystems/topics/financing/healthreport/whr_background/en).

2. *The impact of global crises on health: money, weather and microbe.* Address by Margaret Chan at: 23rd Forum on Global Issues, Berlin, Germany, 2009 (http://www.who.int/dg/speeches/2009/financial_crisis_20090318/en/index.html, accessed 23 June 2010).

3. Witter S. *Summary of position on user fees, selected African and Asian countries (including all PSA countries).* Briefing note for the Department for International Development, 2009 (unpublished).

4. National Health Accounts [online database]. Geneva, World Health Organization (http://www.who.int/nha, accessed 23 June 2010).

5. *Access to health care in Burundi. Results of three epidemiological surveys.* Brussels, Médecins Sans Frontières, 2004 (http://www.msf.org/source/countries/africa/burundi/2004/report/burundi-healthcare.pdf, accessed 25 June 2010).

6. Leive A, Xu K. Coping with out-of-pocket health payments: empirical evidence from 15 African countries. *Bulletin of the World Health Organization*, 2008,86:849-856. doi:10.2471/BLT.07.049403 PMID:19030690

7. McIntyre D et al. What are the economic consequences for households of illness and of paying for health care in low- and middle-income country contexts? *Social Science & Medicine (1982)*, 2006,62:858-865. doi:10.1016/j.socscimed.2005.07.001 PMID:16099574

8. *World report on disability and rehabilitation.* Geneva, World Health Organization (unpublished).

9. Xu K et al. Understanding the impact of eliminating user fees: utilization and catastrophic health expenditures in Uganda. *Social Science & Medicine (1982)*, 2006,62:866-876. doi:10.1016/j.socscimed.2005.07.004 PMID:16139936

10. Habicht J et al. Detecting changes in financial protection: creating evidence for policy in Estonia. *Health Policy and Planning*, 2006,21:421-431. doi:10.1093/heapol/czl026 PMID:16951417

11. Saksena P et al. *Impact of mutual health insurance on access to health care and financial risk protection in Rwanda.* World health report 2010 background paper, no. 6 (http://www.who.int/healthsystems/topics/financing/healthreport/whr_background/en).

12. James CD, Bayarsaikhan D, Bekedam H. Health-financing strategy for WHO's Asia-Pacific Region. *Lancet*, 2010,375:1417-1419. doi:10.1016/S0140-6736(10)60552-1 PMID:20417844

13. *Health financing strategy for the Asia Pacific region (2010–2015).* Manila and New Delhi, World Health Organization, WHO Regional Office for the Western Pacific and WHO Regional Office for South-East Asia, 2009 (http://www.wpro.who.int/internet/resources.ashx/HCF/HCF+strategy+2010-2015.pdf, accessed 25 June 2010).

14. Cohen J, Dupas P. Free distribution or cost-sharing? Evidence from a randomized malaria prevention experiment. *The Quarterly Journal of Economics*, 2010,125:1-45. doi:10.1162/qjec.2010.125.1.1

15. Kremer M, Miguel E. The illusion of sustainability. *The Quarterly Journal of Economics*, 2007,122:1007-1065. doi:10.1162/qjec.122.3.1007

16. Gilson L, McIntyre D. Removing user fees for primary care in Africa: the need for careful action. *BMJ*, 2005,331:762-765. doi:10.1136/bmj.331.7519.762 PMID:16195296

17. Jowett M, Danielyan E. Is there a role for user charges? Thoughts on health system reform in Armenia. *Bulletin of the World Health Organization*, 2010,88:472-473. doi:10.2471/BLT.09.074765 PMID:20539867

18. Gaal P, Cashin C, Shishkin S. Strategies to address informal payments for health care. In: Kutzin J, Cashin C, Jakab M, eds. *Implementing health reform: lessons from countries in transition*. Brussels, European Observatory on Health Systems and Policies, 2010.

19. Kruk ME et al. User fee exemptions are not enough: out-of-pocket payments for 'free' delivery services in rural Tanzania. *Tropical medicine & international health : TM & IH*, 2008,13:1442-1451. doi:10.1111/j.1365-3156.2008.02173.x PMID:18983268

20. Lewis M. Informal payments and the financing of health care in developing and transition countries. *Health Aff (Millwood)*, 2007,26:984-997. doi:10.1377/hlthaff.26.4.984 PMID:17630441

21. *Women and health: today's evidence, tomorrow's agenda.* Geneva, World Health Organization, 2009 (http://whqlibdoc.who.int/publications/2009/9789241563857_eng.pdf, accessed 25 June 2010).

22. Rossi L et al. Evaluation of health, nutrition and food security programmes in a complex emergency: the case of Congo as an example of a chronic post-conflict situation. *Public Health Nutrition*, 2006,9:551-556. doi:10.1079/PHN2005928 PMID:16923285

23. *Global health cluster position paper: removing user fees for primary health care services during humanitarian crises*. Geneva, World Health Organization, 2010 (http://www.who.int/hac/global_health_cluster/about/policy_strategy/EN_final_position_paper_on_user_fees.pdf, accessed 25 June 2010).

24. Andrews S, Mohan S. User charges in health care: some issues. *Economic and Political Weekly*, 2002,37:3793-3795.

25. Akin J, Birdsall N, Ferranti D. *Financing health services in developing countries: an agenda for reform*. Washington, DC, The World Bank, 1987.

26. Resolution AFR/RC37/R6. Women's and children's health through the funding and management of essential drugs at community level: Bamako Initiative. In: *37th Regional Committee, Bamako, 9–16 September 1987*. Brazzaville, World Health Organization Regional Office for Africa, 1987.

27. Waddington C, Enyimayew K. A price to pay, part 2: the impact of user charges in the Volta region of Ghana. *The International Journal of Health Planning and Management*, 1990,5:287-312. doi:10.1002/hpm.4740050405

28. Mwabu G, Mwanzia J, Liambila W. User charges in government health facilities in Kenya: effect on attendance and revenue. *Health Policy and Planning*, 1995,10:164-170. doi:10.1093/heapol/10.2.164 PMID:10143454

29. Knippenberg R et al. *Increasing clients' power to scale up health services for the poor: the Bamako Initiative in West Africa*. Washington, DC, The World Bank, 2003 (http://www-wds.worldbank.org/external/default/WDS-ContentServer/IW3P/IB/2003/10/24/000160016_20031024114304/Rendered/PDF/269540Bamako0Increasing0clients0power.pdf, accessed 25 June 2010).

30. Soucat A et al. Local cost sharing in Bamako Initiative systems in Benin and Guinea: assuring the financial viability of primary health care. *The International Journal of Health Planning and Management*, 1997,12:Suppl 1S109-S135. doi:10.1002/(SICI)1099-1751(199706)12:1+<S109::AID-HPM468>3.3.CO;2-7 PMID:10169906

31. Litvack JI, Bodart C. User fees plus quality equals improved access to health care: results of a field experiment in Cameroon. *Social Science & Medicine (1982)*, 1993,37:369-383. doi:10.1016/0277-9536(93)90267-8 PMID:8356485

32. Batungwanayo C, Reyntjens L. *Impact of the presidential decree for free care on the quality of health care in Burundi*. Buju Burundi, 2006.

33. Witter S, Armar-Klemesu M, Dieng T. National fee exemption schemes for deliveries: comparing the recent experiences of Ghana and Senegal. In: Richard F, Witter S, De Brouwere V, eds. *Reducing financial barriers to obstetric care in low-income countries*. Antwerp, ITGPress, 2008:168–198.

34. Thomson S, Mossialos E. *Primary care and prescription drugs: coverage, cost-sharing, and financial protection in six European countries*. New York, The Commonwealth Fund, 2010 (http://www.commonwealthfund.org/~/media/Files/Publications/Issue%20Brief/2010/Mar/1384_Thomson_primary_care_prescription_drugs_intl_ib_325.pdf, accessed 25 June 2010).

35. Mkandawire T. *Targeting and universalism in poverty reduction*. Geneva, United Nations Research Institute for Social Development, 2005 (http://www.unrisd.org/unrisd/website/document.nsf/462fc27bd1fce00880256b4a0060d2af/955fb8a594eea0b0c12570ff00493eaa/$FILE/mkandatarget.pdf, accessed 25 June 2010).

36. Wilkinson D, Holloway J, Fallavier P. *The impact of user fees on access, equity and health provider practices in Cambodia* (WHO Health Sector Reform Phase III Project Report). Phnom Penh, Cambodian Ministry of Health/Health Economics Task Force, 2001.

37. Hardeman W et al. Access to health care for all? User fees plus a Health Equity Fund in Sotnikum, Cambodia. *Health Policy and Planning*, 2004,19:22-32. doi:10.1093/heapol/czh003 PMID:14679282

38. Noirhomme M et al. Improving access to hospital care for the poor: comparative analysis of four health equity funds in Cambodia. *Health Policy and Planning*, 2007,22:246-262. doi:10.1093/heapol/czm015 PMID:17526640

39. Bigdeli M, Annear PL. Barriers to access and the purchasing function of health equity funds: lessons from Cambodia. *Bulletin of the World Health Organization*, 2009,87:560-564. doi:10.2471/BLT.08.053058 PMID:19649372

40. Kutzin J. *Health expenditures, reforms and policy priorities for the Kyrgyz Republic*. Bishkek, World Health Organization and Ministry of Health, 2003 (Policy Research Paper 24, Manas Health Policy Analysis Project).

41. Bitran R, Giedion U. *Waivers and exemptions for health services in developing countries*. Washington, DC, The World Bank, 2003 (http://info.worldbank.org/etools/docs/library/80083/SouthAsia/southasia/pdf/readings/day1/aldeman.pdf, accessed 25 June 2010).

42. Jacobs B, Price NL, Oeun S. Do exemptions from user fees mean free access to health services? A case study from a rural Cambodian hospital. *Tropical medicine & international health : TM & IH*, 2007,12:1391-1401. PMID:17949399

43. Nishtar S. *Choked pipes: reforming Pakistan's mixed health system*. Oxford, Oxford University Press, 2010.

44. Gotsadze G, Gaal P. Coverage decisions: benefit entitlements and patient cost-sharing. In: Kutzin J, Cashin C, Jakab M, eds. *Implementing health financing reform: lessons from countries in transition*. Brussels, European Observatory on Health Systems and Policies, 2010.

45. Xu K et al. Protecting households from catastrophic health spending. *Health Aff (Millwood)*, 2007,26:972-983. doi:10.1377/hlthaff.26.4.972 PMID:17630440

46. Ridde V, Robert E, Meesen B. *Les pressions exercées par l'abolition du paiement des soins sur les systèmes de santé*. World health report 2010 background paper, no.18 (http://www.who.int/healthsystems/topics/financing/healthreport/whr_background/en).

47. Masiye F et al. *Removal of user fees at primary health care facilities in Zambia: a study of the effects on utilisation and quality of care*. Harare, Regional Network for Equity in Health in east and southern Africa, 2008 (Report No. 57; http://www.equinetafrica.org/bibl/docs/Dis57FINchitah.pdf, accessed 25 June 2010).

48. Nabyonga J et al. Abolition of cost-sharing is pro-poor: evidence from Uganda. *Health Policy and Planning*, 2005,20:100-108. doi:10.1093/heapol/czi012 PMID:15746218

49. *An unnecessary evil? User fees for healthcare in low-income countries*. London, Save the Children Fund, 2005 (http://www.savethechildren.org.uk/en/docs/An_Unnecessary_Evil.pdf, accessed 25 June 2010).

50. *Your money or your life. Will leaders act now to save lives and make health care free in poor countries?* Oxford, Oxfam International, 2009 (http://www.oxfam.org.uk/resources/policy/health/downloads/bp_your_money_%20or_your_life.pdf, accessed 25 June 2010).

51. Nolan B, Turbat V. *Cost recovery in public health services in sub-Saharan Africa*. Washington, DC, The World Bank, 1995.

52. Gilson L, Mills A. Health sector reforms in sub-Saharan Africa: lessons of the last 10 years. *Health Policy*, 1995,32:215-243. doi:10.1016/0168-8510(95)00737-D PMID:10156640

53. Nyonator F, Kutzin J. Health for some? The effects of user fees in the Volta Region of Ghana. *Health Policy and Planning*, 1999,14:329-341. doi:10.1093/heapol/14.4.329 PMID:10787649

54. Witter S et al. Providing free maternal health care: ten lessons from an evaluation of the national delivery exemption policy in Ghana. *Global Health Action*, 2009,2: PMID:20027275

55. Xu K et al. Understanding the impact of eliminating user fees: utilization and catastrophic health expenditures in Uganda. *Social Science & Medicine (1982)*, 2006,62:866-876. doi:10.1016/j.socscimed.2005.07.004 PMID:16139936

56. Gaal P, Jakab M, Shishkin S. Strategies to address informal payments for health care. In: Kutzin J, Cashin C, Jakab M, eds. *Implementing health financing reform: lessons from countries in transition*. Brussels, European Observatory on Health Policies and Systems, 2010.

57. Yates R. Universal health care and the removal of user fees. *Lancet*, 2009,373:2078-2081. doi:10.1016/S0140-6736(09)60258-0 PMID:19362359

58. Busse R, Schreyögg J, Gericke C. *Analyzing changes in health financing arrangements in high-income countries: a comprehensive framework approach*. Washington, DC, The World Bank, 2007 (Health, Nutrition and Population Discussion Paper; http://go.worldbank.org/LSI0CP39O0, accessed 25 June 2010).

59. Kwon S. Healthcare financing reform and the new single payer system in the Republic of Korea: Social solidarity or efficiency? *International Social Security Review*, 2003,56:75-94. doi:10.1111/1468-246X.00150

60. What? No waiting lists? *Bulletin of the World Health Organization*, 2010,88:241-320. doi:10.2471/BLT.10.000410

61. Van de Ven WPMM, Schut FT. Managed competition in the Netherlands: still work-in-progress. *Health Economics*, 2009,18:253-255. doi:10.1002/hec.1446 PMID:19206093

62. Towse A, Mills A, Tangcharoensathien V. Learning from Thailand's health reforms. *BMJ*, 2004,328:103-105. doi:10.1136/bmj.328.7431.103 PMID:14715608

63. Smith PC. *Formula funding of health services: learning from experience in some developed countries*. Geneva, World Health Organization, 2008 (HSS/HSF/DP.08.1).

64. Devadasan N et al. The landscape of community health insurance in India: an overview based on 10 case studies. *Health Policy*, 2006,78:224-234. doi:10.1016/j.healthpol.2005.10.005 PMID:16293339

65. Fonteneau B, Galland B. The community-based model: mutual health organizations in Africa. In: Churchill C, ed. *Protecting the poor: a microinsurance compendium*. Geneva, International Labour Organization, 2006.

66. Bennett S, Creese A, Monasch R. *Health insurance schemes for people outside formal sector employment*. Geneva, World Health Organization, 1998 (WHO/ARA/97.13).

67. Letourmy A, Pavy-Letourmy A. *La micro-assurance de santé dans les pays à faible revenu*. Paris, Agence française de Développement, 2005.

68. Lekhan V, Rudiy V, Shishkin S. *The Ukrainian health financing system and options for reform.* Copenhagen, World Health Organization Regional Office for Europe, 2007 (http://www.euro.who.int/__data/assets/pdf_file/0007/97423/E90754.pdf, accessed 25 June 2010).

69. Criel B et al. Community health insurance in developing countries. In: Carrin G et al. eds. *Health systems policy, finance and organization.* Amsterdam, Elsevier, 2009.

70. Soors W et al. *Community health insurance and universal coverage: multiple paths, many rivers to cross.* World health report 2010 background paper, no. 48 (http://www.who.int/healthsystems/topics/financing/healthreport/whr_background/en).

71. Tangcharoensathien V et al. *Achieving universal coverage in Thailand: what lessons do we learn? A case study commissioned by the Health Systems Knowledge Network.* Geneva, World Health Organization, 2007.

72. Donaldson D, Pannarunothai S, Tangcharoensathien V. Health financing in Thailand technical report. Management Sciences for Health and Health Systems Research Institute. Manila, Asian Development Bank, Thailand Health Management and Financing Study Project, 1999.

73. Tangcharoensathien V et al. *Universal coverage scheme in Thailand: equity outcomes and future agendas to meet challenges.* World health report 2010 background paper, no. 43 (http://www.who.int/healthsystems/topics/financing/healthreport/whr_background/en).

74. Hrobon P, Machacek T, Julinek T. *Healthcare reform in the Czech Republic in the 21st century Europe.* Prague, Health Reform CZ, 2005 (http://healthreform.cz/content/files/en/Reform/1_Publications/EN_publikace.pdf, accessed 24 June 2010).

75. Jeong H-S. *Expanding insurance coverage to informal sector population: experience from the Republic of Korea.* World health report 2010 background paper, no. 38 (http://www.who.int/healthsystems/topics/financing/healthreport/whr_background/en).

76. Xu K et al. *Financial risk protection of national health insurance in the Republic of Korea: 1995–2007.* World health report 2010 background paper, no. 23 (http://www.who.int/healthsystems/topics/financing/healthreport/whr_background/en).

77. Frenk J. Comprehensive policy analysis for health system reform. *Health Policy*, 1995,32:257-277. doi:10.1016/0168-8510(95)00739-F PMID:10156642

78. Lloyd-Sherlock P. When social health insurance goes wrong: lessons from Argentina and Mexico. *Social Policy and Administration*, 2006,40:353-368. doi:10.1111/j.1467-9515.2006.00494.x

79. Savedoff WD. Is there a case for social insurance? *Health Policy and Planning*, 2004,19:183-184. doi:10.1093/heapol/czh022 PMID:15070867

80. Londoño JL, Frenk J. Structured pluralism: towards an innovative model for health system reform in Latin America. *Health Policy*, 1997,41:1-36. doi:10.1016/S0168-8510(97)00010-9 PMID:10169060

81. Kutzin J et al. Reforms in the pooling of funds. In: Kutzin J, Cashin C, Jakab M, eds. *Implementing health financing reform: lessons from countries in transition.* Brussels, European Observatory on Health Policies and Systems, 2010.

82. Knaul FM, Frenk J. Health insurance in Mexico: achieving universal coverage through structural reform. *Health Aff (Millwood)*, 2005,24:1467-1476. doi:10.1377/hlthaff.24.6.1467 PMID:16284018

83. James C, Savedoff WD. *Risk pooling and redistribution in health care: an empirical analysis of attitudes toward solidarity.* World health report 2010 background paper, no. 5 (http://www.who.int/healthsystems/topics/financing/healthreport/whr_background/en).

84. Xu K et al. *Exploring the thresholds of health expenditure for protection against financial risk.* World health report 2010 background paper, no. 19 (http://www.who.int/healthsystems/topics/financing/healthreport/whr_background/en).

85. Interview with Dr Mirta Roses Periago, Director of the Pan American Health Organization. International Food Policy Research Institute. IFPRI Forum, Online Edition 15 December 2009 (http://ifpriforum.wordpress.com/2009/12/15/interview-roses-periago/, accessed 24 June 2010).

86. *Towards the fifth summit of the Americas: regional challenges.* Washington, DC, Organization of American States, undated (http://www.summit-americas.org/pubs/towards_v_summit_regional_challenges_en.pdf accessed 24 June 2010).

87. Jowett M, Shishkin S. *Extending population coverage in the national health insurance scheme in the Republic of Moldova.* Copenhagen, World Health Organization Regional Office for Europe, 2010 (http://www.euro.who.int/__data/assets/pdf_file/0005/79295/E93573.pdf, accessed 24 June 2010).

88. Shishkin S, Kacevicus G, Ciocanu M. *Evaluation of Moldova's 2004 health financing reform.* Copenhagen, World Health Organization Regional Office for Europe, 2008 (http://www.euro.who.int/__data/assets/pdf_file/0008/78974/HealthFin_Moldova.pdf, accessed 24 June 2010).

89. Kutzin J, Jakab M, Shishkin S. From scheme to system: social health insurance funds and the transformation of health financing in Kyrgyzstan and Moldova. *Advances in Health Economics and Health Services Research*, 2009,21:291-312. PMID:19791707

90. Kutzin J et al. Reforms in the pooling of funds. In: Kutzin J, Cashin C, Jakab M, eds. *Implementing health financing reform: lessons from countries in transition*. Copenhagen, World Health Organization Regional Office for Europe and the European Observatory on Health Policies and Systems, 2010.

91. Schmidt U. Shepherding major health system reforms: a conversation with German health minister Ulla Schmidt. Interview by Tsung-Mei Cheng and Uwe Reinhardt. *Health Aff (Millwood)*, 2008,27:w204-w213. doi:10.1377/hlthaff.27.3.w204 PMID:18397935

92. Ognyanova D, Busse R. Health fund now operational. *Health Policy Monitor*, May 2009 (http://www.hpm.org/survey/de/a13/3).

93. Goudge J et al. Affordability, availability and acceptability barriers to health care for the chronically ill: longitudinal case studies from South Africa. *BMC Health Services Research*, 2009,9:75- doi:10.1186/1472-6963-9-75 PMID:19426533

94. James CD et al. To retain or remove user fees?: reflections on the current debate in low- and middle-income countries. *Applied Health Economics and Health Policy*, 2006,5:137-153. doi:10.2165/00148365-200605030-00001 PMID:17132029

95. Saksena P et al. *Health services utilization and out-of-pocket expenditure in public and private facilities in low-income countries*. World health report 2010 background paper, no. 20 (http://www.who.int/healthsystems/topics/financing/healthreport/whr_background/en).

96. Ensor T, Cooper S. Overcoming barriers to health service access: influencing the demand side. *Health Policy and Planning*, 2004,19:69-79. doi:10.1093/heapol/czh009 PMID:14982885

97. Saksena P et al. Patient costs for paediatric hospital admissions in Tanzania: a neglected burden? *Health Policy and Planning*, 2010,25:328-333. doi:10.1093/heapol/czq003 PMID:20129938

98. Goudge J et al. The household costs of health care in rural South Africa with free public primary care and hospital exemptions for the poor. *Tropical medicine & international health : TM & IH*, 2009,14:458-467. doi:10.1111/j.1365-3156.2009.02256.x PMID:19254274

99. Prakongsai P, Limwattananon S, Tangcharoensathien V. The equity impact of the universal coverage policy: lessons from Thailand. *Advances in Health Economics and Health Services Research*, 2009,21:57-81. PMID:19791699

100. Gupta I, William J, Shalini R. *Demand side financing in health. How far can it address the issue of low utilization in developing countries?* World health report 2010 background paper, no. 27) (http://www.who.int/healthsystems/topics/financing/healthreport/whr_background/en).

101. Ensor T. *Consumer-led demand side financing for health and education: an international review*. Dhaka, World Health Organization Bangladesh Country Office, 2003 (WHO/BAN/DSF/03.1) (http://www.whoban.org/dsf_international_review.pdf, accessed 25 June 2010).

102. Doetinchem O, Xu K, Carrin G. *Conditional cash transfers: what's in it for health?* Geneva, World Health Organization, 2008 (WHO/HSS/HSF/PB/08.01).

103. Rawlings LB. Evaluating the impact of conditional cash transfer programs *The World Bank Research Observer*, 2005,20:29-55. doi:10.1093/wbro/lki001

104. Leroy JL, Ruel M, Verhofstadt E. The impact of conditional cash transfer programmes on child nutrition: a review of evidence using a programme theory framework. *Journal of Development Effectiveness*, 2009,1:103-129. doi:10.1080/19439340902924043

105. Fernald LC, Gertler PJ, Neufeld LM. Role of cash in conditional cash transfer programmes for child health, growth, and development: an analysis of Mexico's Oportunidades. *Lancet*, 2008,371:828-837. doi:10.1016/S0140-6736(08)60382-7 PMID:18328930

106. Barham T.. A healthier start: the effect of conditional cash transfers on neonatal and infant mortality in rural Mexico. *Journal of Development Economics*, In press, corrected proof available doi:10.1016/j.jdeveco.2010.01.003.

Chapter 4 | More health for the money

Key messages

- All countries can do something, many of them a great deal, to improve the efficiency of their health systems, thereby releasing resources that could be used to cover more people, more services and/or more of the costs.

- Some of these actions would aim to improve efficiency in a particular area of the health system, such as medicines. Others would address the incentives inherent in the health financing system; in particular, how services are bought and providers paid.

- All countries can look to improve efficiency by taking a more strategic approach when providing or buying health services, e.g. decide which services to purchase based on information on the health needs of the population and link payments to providers on their performance and to information on service costs, quality and impact.

- All provider payment mechanisms have strengths and weaknesses, but particular care should be taken with fee-for-service payments, which offer incentives to over-service those people who can pay or who are covered from pooled funds, and to underservice those who cannot pay.

- Reducing fragmentation in the flow and pooling of funds for health and in service delivery will also increase efficiency.

- There is no convincing evidence that private-sector health facilities are more, or less, efficient than government facilities. It depends on the setting.

- By setting rules and ensuring they are followed, effective governance is the key to improving efficiency and equity.

- Donors can also contribute by helping to develop domestic financing institutions and by reducing the fragmented way their funds are delivered and countries are asked to report on their use. They could also reduce duplication at the global level.

4

More health for the money

Using resources wisely

Health-care systems haemorrhage money. A recent study by the PricewaterhouseCoopers' Health Research Institute estimated that more than half of the US$ 2 trillion-plus that the United States of America spends on health each year is wasted; a Thomson-Reuters study reported a lower but still substantial figure of US$ 600–850 billion per year (1, 2). The European Health care Fraud and Corruption Network says that of the annual global health expenditure of about US$ 5.3 trillion, a little less than 6%, or about US$ 300 billion, is lost to mistakes or corruption alone (3).

While some countries lose more than others, most, if not all, fail to fully exploit the resources available, whether through poorly executed procurement, irrational medicine use, misallocated and mismanaged human and technical resources or fragmented financing and administration. But there is nothing inevitable about this and there are many shades of inefficiency. Some countries obtain higher levels of coverage and better health outcomes for their money than others, and the gap between what countries achieve and what they could potentially achieve with the same resources is sometimes enormous (4). This is illustrated in Fig. 4.1, where substantial variations in the proportion of births attended by skilled health workers is shown, even for countries with similar total health expenditures.

While raising more money for health is crucial for lower-income countries striving to move closer to universal coverage, it is just as important to get the most out of the resources available. Finding the most efficient ways to meet the multiple challenges health systems face is also an issue for those countries that might be struggling to sustain high levels of coverage in the face of constantly increasing costs and growing demand.

There are many opportunities for efficiency gains. This does not mean simply cutting costs. Efficiency, as we will discuss in the following pages, is a measure of the quality and/or quantity of output (i.e. health outcomes or services) for a given level of input (i.e. cost). So efficiency gains could help to contain costs – an important objective in many countries – by reducing the costs of service delivery. However, no one wants to contain costs by reducing health outcomes, so seeking efficiency gains should also be seen as a means of extending coverage for the same cost.

How countries can improve the efficiency of their health-care systems is the subject of this chapter.

Ten leading causes of inefficiency

Every country can improve efficiency and in so doing, advance the cause of universal health coverage. Table 4.1 identifies 10 problem areas and suggests ways to make health systems more efficient.

Eliminate unnecessary spending on medicines

Medicines account for 20–30% of global health spending, slightly more in low- and middle-income countries, and, therefore, constitute a major part of the budget of whoever is paying for health services (7). In many cases that burden would be lighter if governments and individuals were paying a fair price. But what exactly is a fair price? International reference prices are a useful starting point for procurement officers in their negotiations. These are determined by calculating the median paid for the same medicine in comparable countries (8). Without such cross-country price information, buyers can struggle to obtain a fair deal in a global pharmaceuticals market that is neither transparent nor efficient, and where there is an enormous range in the prices paid for identical products. A recent medicine pricing study revealed that while generic medicines in the WHO regions of the Americas, South-East Asia and the Eastern Mediterranean were bought by the public sector at close to international reference prices, in the African, European and Western Pacific Regions, governments paid an average 34–44% more than they needed to (Fig. 4.2) (9).

The same study revealed that certain medicines are nearly always sold at substantial mark ups, with the prices varying significantly from country to country. Procurement prices for the branded form of ciprofloxacin (a broad spectrum antibiotic), for example, vary widely across developing countries, with some paying up to 67 times the international reference price (9). Even in high-income countries, there is considerable pricing variability. In the USA, branded ciprofloxacin is reported to sell for between US$ 90 and US$ 100 per course of treatment; it sells for half that price in the United Kingdom (10).

Buying branded formulations rather than generic ones also drives inefficiency. A recent study covering 18 medicines in 17 largely middle-income countries revealed that

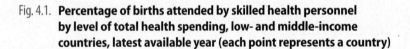

Fig. 4.1. **Percentage of births attended by skilled health personnel by level of total health spending, low- and middle-income countries, latest available year (each point represents a country)**

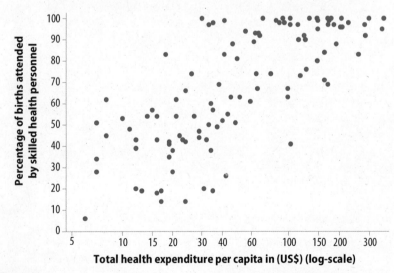

Source: (5).

Table 4.1. **Ten leading sources of inefficiency**

Source of inefficiency	Common reasons for inefficiency	Ways to address inefficiency
1. Medicines: underuse of generics and higher than necessary prices for medicines	Inadequate controls on supply-chain agents, prescribers and dispensers; lower perceived efficacy/safety of generic medicines; historical prescribing patterns and inefficient procurement/distribution systems; taxes and duties on medicines; excessive mark-ups.	Improve prescribing guidance, information, training and practice. Require, permit or offer incentives for generic substitution. Develop active purchasing based on assessment of costs and benefits of alternatives. Ensure transparency in purchasing and tenders. Remove taxes and duties. Control excessive mark-ups. Monitor and publicize medicine prices.
2. Medicines: use of substandard and counterfeit medicines	Inadequate pharmaceutical regulatory structures/mechanisms; weak procurement systems.	Strengthen enforcement of quality standards in the manufacture of medicines; carry out product testing; enhance procurement systems with pre-qualification of suppliers.
3. Medicines: inappropriate and ineffective use	Inappropriate prescriber incentives and unethical promotion practices; consumer demand/expectations; limited knowledge about therapeutic effects; inadequate regulatory frameworks.	Separate prescribing and dispensing functions; regulate promotional activities; improve prescribing guidance, information, training and practice; disseminate public information.
4. Health-care products and services: overuse or supply of equipment, investigations and procedures	Supplier-induced demand; fee-for-service payment mechanisms; fear of litigation (defensive medicine).	Reform incentive and payment structures (e.g. capitation or diagnosis-related group); develop and implement clinical guidelines.
5. Health workers: inappropriate or costly staff mix, unmotivated workers	Conformity with pre-determined human resource policies and procedures; resistance by medical profession; fixed/inflexible contracts; inadequate salaries; recruitment based on favouritism.	Undertake needs-based assessment and training; revise remuneration policies; introduce flexible contracts and/or performance-related pay; implement task-shifting and other ways of matching skills to needs.
6. Health-care services: inappropriate hospital admissions and length of stay	Lack of alternative care arrangements; insufficient incentives to discharge; limited knowledge of best practice.	Provide alternative care (e.g. day care); alter incentives to hospital providers; raise knowledge about efficient admission practice.
7. Health-care services: inappropriate hospital size (low use of infrastructure)	Inappropriate level of managerial resources for coordination and control; too many hospitals and inpatient beds in some areas, not enough in others. Often this reflects a lack of planning for health service infrastructure development.	Incorporate inputs and output estimation into hospital planning; match managerial capacity to size; reduce excess capacity to raise occupancy rate to 80–90% (while controlling length of stay).
8. Health-care services: medical errors and suboptimal quality of care	Insufficient knowledge or application of clinical-care standards and protocols; lack of guidelines; inadequate supervision.	Improve hygiene standards in hospitals; provide more continuity of care; undertake more clinical audits; monitor hospital performance.
9. Health system leakages: waste, corruption and fraud	Unclear resource allocation guidance; lack of transparency; poor accountability and governance mechanisms; low salaries.	Improve regulation/governance, including strong sanction mechanisms; assess transparency/vulnerability to corruption; undertake public spending tracking surveys; promote codes of conduct.
10. Health interventions: inefficient mix/inappropriate level of strategies	Funding high-cost, low-effect interventions when low-cost, high-impact options are unfunded. Inappropriate balance between levels of care, and/or between prevention, promotion and treatment.	Regular evaluation and incorporation into policy of evidence on the costs and impact of interventions, technologies, medicines, and policy options.

Source (6).

costs to patients could be reduced by an average of 60% by switching from originator brands to the lowest priced generic equivalents (*11*). For this group of countries, this represents a total saving of US$ 155 million for this limited basket of medicines alone.

The global gains from a more systematic use of generics might be even larger in some high-income countries. For example, France has implemented a strategy of generic substitution and it has been estimated that the wider use of generics saved €1.32 billion in 2008 alone, which was the equivalent then of US$ 1.94 billion (*12, 13*).

Improve quality control for medicines

Whether substandard, spurious, falsified, falsely labelled, counterfeit or expired, "bad" medicines are too expensive at any price, and avoiding them is another way to stop wasting resources. More than half the products circulating in South-East Asia supposedly containing the anti-malarial artesunate are reported to contain no active ingredient (*14*), while a study of three African countries reported that 26–44% of the samples of antimalarial medicines failed quality tests (*15*).

There is little reliable information to allow an estimate of the extent of the problem. However, the United States Food and Drug Administration estimated that counterfeit products account for more than 10% of the global medicines market; if we use this as a lower limit, annual global earnings from the sales of substandard medicines would be more than US$ 32 billion (*16*). That is US$ 32 billion of health spending that might generate little health improvement.

Countries seeking to eliminate bad products have several options, notably, adhering to good manufacturing practices (GMP) in producing pharmaceuticals and buying from GMP producers. GMP are designed to ensure that products are consistently produced and controlled according to a specific set of quality standards to avoid contamination, incorrect labelling and inappropriate levels of active ingredient (*17*). Many countries have formulated their own requirements for GMP based on the model developed by WHO, while others have adapted requirements already in place.

To aid access to medicines that meet unified standards of quality, safety and efficacy for HIV/AIDS, malaria, tuberculosis and reproductive health, WHO

Fig. 4.2. **Median price ratios of public-sector procurement prices for generic medicines,ª by WHO region**

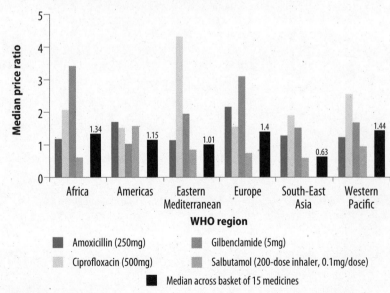

ª Ratio of the median procurement price to the international reference price of the Management Sciences for Health.
Source: (*9*).

set up a prequalification programme in 2001. It was intended to support United Nations procurement agencies but, over time, the list of prequalified medicines has become a resource for anyone bulk-buying medicines, including national procurement agencies (*18*).

Use medicines appropriately

The irrational use of medicines not only leads to suffering and death, it draws resources away from effective, evidence-based interventions. Despite the fact that many countries have adopted national medicines policies and essential medicines programmes that encourage appropriate use, fewer than half of all patients treated in low- and middle-income countries receive care according to clinical guidelines for common diseases in primary care (*19*). It is estimated that more than half of all medicines globally are prescribed, dispensed or sold inappropriately (*19*), and that half of all patients fail to take their medication as prescribed or dispensed (*20*). Irrational use may take many forms, including the use of harmful medicine mixtures (polypharmacy), the overuse of antibiotics and injections, failure to prescribe in accordance with clinical guidelines, or inappropriate self-medication (*21*).

Overuse and misuse of antibiotics is a particularly serious global problem, with two thirds of all antibiotics being sold without prescription through unregulated private markets. Many patients are prescribed incorrect or inadequate doses or fail to complete the course prescribed. Fewer than half of all patients with acute diarrhoea obtain treatment with cheap and extremely effective oral rehydration salts, while more than half are given expensive and – for this purpose – useless antibiotics. As an example, the overuse of antibiotics to treat acute respiratory tract infections in low- and middle-income countries is estimated to add an average 36% to the cost of care (*22*).

Get the most out of technologies and services

Medical technologies can be crucial to providing good health services, provided they are selected and used properly, based on scientific evidence and best practice (*23*). Too often procurement policy is distorted by the marketing pressure of equipment manufacturers. This is as true for high- as it is for low-income countries, perhaps more so given the greater scope for spending. Modern medical technology is a major contributor to rising costs in Organization for Economic Co-operation and Development (OECD) countries and the extent to which any particular country embraces it is not always based on need. Among OECD countries, the highest number of magnetic resonance imaging (MRI) and *computed tomography* (CT) scanners per capita is found in Japan, while the USA leads the world in diagnostic imaging referrals: 91.2 MRI examinations per 1000 of population (compared with an OECD average of 41.3 per 1000); and 227.8 CT scans per 1000 (compared with an OECD average of 110) (*24*). A significant proportion of these tests are believed to be medically unnecessary.

Unnecessary purchase and use of equipment can also occur in low-income countries, but generally speaking, resource-poor settings have other technology challenges. It is estimated that at least 50% of medical equipment in developing countries is either partly usable or totally unusable (25). In subSaharan Africa, up to 70% of medical equipment stands idle. Studies suggest there are several reasons for this type of broad systemic failure, including mismanagement of the technology acquisition process, and a lack of user training and effective technical support (26). Where medical technology is available for use, it is too often the cause of substandard or hazardous diagnosis, or treatment that can pose a threat to the safety of patients. Inappropriate medical technology also imposes a financial burden on systems that can ill afford it.

Ironically, one of the biggest causes of inefficiency as it relates to medical technologies in low-income countries is donations. In some countries, almost 80% of health-care equipment comes from international donors or foreign governments, much of it remaining idle for various reasons. A recent study carried out in the West Bank and Gaza Strip offers an example (27). Large consignments of such equipment were sent to the Gaza Strip after hostilities ended in January 2009. While some of the donated equipment was useful, a significant proportion could not be integrated into the health-care system and sat in warehouses.

This type of problem could be avoided if development partners consulted with recipient countries to clarify their needs and capacities to service donated equipment. It is also incumbent on recipient governments to establish rational management systems, organizing the storage of medical devices by type, model and manufacturer, and checking each donated item for completeness, compatibility and quality.

What applies to technologies also applies to health services. A study comparing the services obtained by patients under the Medicare programme in the USA concluded that "residents in high-spending regions received 60% more care but did not have lower mortality rates, better functional status or higher satisfaction" (28, 29). The differences in practice patterns could not be attributed to differences in medical need and about 30% of the costs of treatment could have been saved if the providers generating high spending reduced their provision of services to the levels found in safe, but conservative treatment regions (30). Similar variations in practice patterns have been found in many countries, indicating similar opportunities for reducing costs and improving efficiency (31–34).

While it is often difficult to establish the precise need for a medical intervention at the individual level, policy-makers can monitor variations in practice patterns within a country, focusing on providers or institutions that provide a large number of services compared with others, or those that provide comparatively few. Reducing this variation can both save resources and improve health outcomes.

Motivate people

Health workers are at the core of a health system and typically account for about half of all health spending in a country (35). While a shortage of health workers is often a major obstacle to strengthening health systems, ineffective recruiting, inappropriate training, poor supervision and maldistribution within countries also undermine efficiency, while inadequate compensation drives excessive turnover or attrition (36). The inevitable result of these compounded failings is reduced productivity and performance.

But exactly how much is lost to workforce inefficiency? Without reliable comprehensive data, it is hard to be precise, but there have been several attempts to measure health-worker productivity in specific contexts. In the United Republic of Tanzania, for example, unexplained absences plus time spent on breaks, on social contacts and on waiting for patients has been reported to reduce productivity levels by 26% (37). In Brazil, Sousa et al. found that the efficiency with which health workers achieve coverage of antenatal care across municipalities in Brazil ranged from less than 20% to more than 95% (38).

Taking admittedly limited examples as indicative of global trends and applying a conservative average level of reported inefficiency (15–25%) to the proportion of total health spending on human resources (45–65%, depending on world income region), it is possible to arrive at a worldwide workforce inefficiency cost that exceeds US$ 500 billion annually.

How to reduce that loss – how to improve the productivity and performance of health workers – is analysed in *The world health report 2006*, which highlighted, among other things, the importance of adequate remuneration and better matching of skills to tasks (36). The matter of provider payment and payment for performance is further discussed below.

Improve hospital efficiency – size and length of stay

In many countries, hospital care absorbs more than half and up to two thirds of total government spending on health, with (often excessive) inpatient admissions and length of stay being significant categories of outlay. Four separate studies of adult inpatients in Canada's health system, for example, found that 24–90% of admissions and 27–66% of inpatient days were inappropriate (39).

Another source of inefficiency is the inappropriate size of some facilities and the range of services they offer. While it might make economic sense to enlarge the size and scope of a hospital to fully exploit available expertise, infrastructure and equipment, there is a point at which efficiency starts to decline. Similarly, small hospitals become inefficient where the fixed infrastructure and administrative costs are shared across too small a caseload, thereby pushing up the cost of an average hospital episode. Research mainly in the USA and the United Kingdom indicates that inefficiencies start below about 200 beds and above 600 (40). A good indicator of hospital efficiency is the use of inpatient facilities as measured by capacity rates. A WHO study of 18 low- and middle-income countries revealed that in district hospitals only 55% of beds were occupied on average, well below the recommended level of 80–90% (6).

A recent review of more than 300 studies looking at the efficiency and productivity of health-care delivery found that hospital efficiency, on average, was about 85%, meaning the hospitals could achieve 15% more than they do for the same cost, or the same levels of service at a 15% reduction in cost (41). No substantial difference was reported between hospitals in the USA, Europe and other parts of the world, although interestingly, public hospitals proved more efficient than both private for-profit and private not-for-profit hospitals (Box 4.1). Applying a median inefficiency rate of 15% to the proportion of total health spending consumed by hospitals in each world income region, almost US$ 300 billion is lost annually to hospital-related inefficiency.

Get care right the first time

Medical error costs money as well as causing suffering. Because of the lack of reliable epidemiological data, the prevalence and magnitude of medical error globally is unknown, but estimates suggest that as many as one in 10 patients in developed countries is harmed while receiving hospital care; in developing countries the number may be significantly higher (49). At any given time, 1.4 million people worldwide suffer from infections acquired in hospitals (50). What this costs health authorities is unknown, but a study in 1999 suggested that preventable medical errors might be killing as many as 98 000 people a year in the USA, at a cost of US$ 17–29 billion (51).

One simple measure to reduce medical error is to encourage hand hygiene. Another is to promote safe injection practices. A third is to ensure accurate diagnostics.

A simple life-saving procedure is the use of checklists, such as the one advocated in WHO's Safe Surgery Saves Lives initiative. Striking results have already been achieved with checklists, notably in Michigan, USA, where a state-wide initiative sought to reduce catheter-associated bloodstream infections by instituting a short checklist. Among other things, the checklist empowered nurses to ensure that doctors were following procedure (52). Bloodstream infections across the participating intensive care units dropped to 1.4 per 1000 days of catheter use, less than 20% of the rate before implementation, saving an estimated 1800 lives over four years. Checklist initiatives can now be found in several countries, including China, Jordan, Thailand, and the United Kingdom.

A more punitive (and potentially controversial) approach to reducing medical errors is to withhold payment for mistakes. This approach is being tested in the USA, where, since October 2008, Medicare, the government-administered social insurance programme providing

---

Box 4.1. The relative efficiency of public and private service delivery

The relative roles of the public and private (for-profit or not-for-profit) sectors in health-care provision have evolved over time and have continued to engender strong debate on ideological grounds. Ultimately, empirical evidence should assist in determining what type of institution most efficiently provides specific services.

Most available studies have focused on the efficiency of hospitals, responsible for about 45–69% of government health spending in subSaharan Africa (42). Hollingsworth (41) recently conducted a meta-analysis of 317 published works on efficiency measures and concluded that, if anything, "public provision may be potentially more efficient than private." However, country studies suggest that the impact of ownership on efficiency is mixed. Lee et al. (43) determined that non-profit hospitals in the USA were more efficient than for-profit hospitals. On the other hand, Swiss hospital efficiency levels did not vary according to ownership (44, 45). In Germany, some studies found private hospitals less technically efficient than publicly owned hospitals, others concluded the inverse, while yet others found no difference at all (46, 47).

There is a dearth of studies measuring the relative efficiencies of public and private health facilities in low- and middle-income countries. Masiye (48) is perhaps the only study that has reported on the significantly positive effect of private ownership on efficiency in Zambian hospitals (mean efficiency for private hospitals was 73% compared with 63% for public hospitals).

This emphasizes that it is unsafe to generalize about which ownership model is best across countries. At the same time, the evidence shows that average levels of efficiency are substantially lower than they could be in all types of hospitals. Hospitals can become more efficient, regardless of ownership, by reducing waste and producing cost-effective interventions. To ensure this happens requires strong government stewardship to set and enforce the rules of operation.

health coverage to people aged 65-plus, has ceased to reimburse hospitals for so-called never-events, those medical errors it deems "reasonably preventable." These include major mistakes, such as operating on the wrong body part, but also complications such as severe bedsores, and certain injuries caused by patient falls. By refusing to pay for mistakes, Medicare hopes to reduce the estimated 98 000 deaths that occur each a year due to medical errors (53).

Eliminate waste and corruption

An estimated 10–25% of public spending on health linked to procurement – buying the necessary inputs such as medicines, equipment and infrastructure – is lost each year to corrupt practices (54). In developed countries alone, fraud and other forms of abuse in health care have been estimated to cost individual governments as much as US$ 12–23 billion per year (55). Because the production and distribution of medicines is a complex multiphase process, there are particular opportunities for many abuses in this area, although the problem extends to all areas of procurement.

Experience has shown that to significantly curb corruption in buying and distributing medicines, two complementary strategies need to be applied: first, a discipline approach that tends to be top-down and based on legislative reforms, establishing the laws, administrative structures and processes needed to ensure transparent medicine regulation and procurement; and second, a more bottom-up values approach that promotes institutional integrity through moral values and principles, and tries to motivate ethical conduct by public servants.

Since 2004, 26 countries have introduced good governance for medicines programmes based on these principles, resulting in a reduction in spending on medicines (56). The Medicines Transparency Alliance is another initiative that focuses on affordability and availability of good-quality medicines through country-level actions that promote efficiencies in the drug-purchasing chain, notably through transparency and accountability (57).

These principles, however, are not limited to buying and distributing medicines, and can be applied to all activities in health. They are underpinned by the core principles of good government, which include accountability, transparency and respect for the rule of law (58). Core regulatory functions that can effectively combat budgetary and other leakages range from registering, accrediting and licensing health providers, facilities and products (to improve quality), to internal oversight and audit functions. Improved governance also requires intelligence and better use of information, so that breaches of practice can be identified and changes monitored.

Critically assess which services are needed

The cost of gaining one healthy year of life has been estimated to range from less than US$ 10 to more than US$ 100 000, depending on the intervention (59, 60). Put another way, if you choose an intervention costing US$ 10 per healthy year of life saved, you can save 100 000 years for US$ 1 million. If you choose the US$ 100 000 intervention, you save only 10 healthy years.

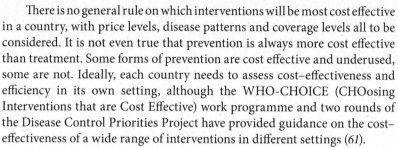

There is no general rule on which interventions will be most cost effective in a country, with price levels, disease patterns and coverage levels all to be considered. It is not even true that prevention is always more cost effective than treatment. Some forms of prevention are cost effective and underused, some are not. Ideally, each country needs to assess cost–effectiveness and efficiency in its own setting, although the WHO-CHOICE (CHOosing Interventions that are Cost Effective) work programme and two rounds of the Disease Control Priorities Project have provided guidance on the cost–effectiveness of a wide range of interventions in different settings (61).

What is clear, however, is that for a variety of reasons, high-cost, low-impact interventions tend to be overused while low-cost, high-impact interventions are underexploited (59, 60). Switching resources from the former to the latter is, therefore, an obvious way to achieve greater efficiencies. Our review of the few studies that compare the status quo with a potentially more appropriate mix of interventions for particular disease complexes or conditions (Table 4.2) suggests that the same health gains could have been obtained with between 16% and 99% of current spending depending on the condition. These savings could then make important contributions to improving health in other ways.

Even allowing for the transaction costs of making the necessary reallocations, the evidence of Table 4.2 suggests that efficiency gains of about 20% would be feasible in countries that prioritize cost-effective interventions. The cost-effective interventions differ, obviously, by country, but in low-income settings, many of the most cost-effective interventions – preventive care and treatment for maternal and neonatal health, or basic childhood vaccinations – are not yet fully implemented, at great cost in human life.

Cost–effectiveness is not the only consideration when deciding on an optimal mix of interventions. In cases where fairness, equity or basic decency are at issue, the social value of a particular health intervention may differ from the value of the health benefits it produces. Consider end-of-life care. It is expensive: in the USA, for example, care during the last year of a patient's life accounts for almost one third of annual Medicare spending, despite these patients accounting for only 5% of enrolments (68). Social values rather than cost–effectiveness considerations determine that societies will continue to provide end-of-life care. A less extreme example, but one often confronting policy-makers in low- and middle-income settings, is the diminishing cost–effectiveness of extending coverage of interventions to remote rural areas. As stated in Chapter 1, the commitment to universal coverage depends to a significant degree on social solidarity, a readiness to make choices that balance efficiency and equity.

While considerations of equity are paramount, it is crucial that governments continue to focus on cost–effectiveness so that they can engage in more active purchasing of services to ensure that the system obtains the best value for money. This is further discussed later in the chapter.

The potential benefits of improving efficiency

By taking the average levels of inefficiency identified in the earlier sections and multiplying them by the average proportions of total health spending associated with each component, it is possible to understand what might be gained through greater efficiency (Table 4.3). The 10 common causes of inefficiency are grouped in this table into five broad categories: human resources for health; medicines; hospitals; leakages due to corruption and waste; and intervention mix.

It is apparent from the table that low-income countries could save annually 12–24% of their total health spending by improving hospital or workforce efficiency, thereby freeing resources to potentially extend financial risk protection to more people or expand the services available. What exactly would happen if countries worked on all these sources of inefficiency at the same time is unclear, but gains would certainly not be totally additive, since an improvement in efficiency of health workers, for example, would also automatically be felt as an improvement in hospital efficiency. A conservative estimate suggests 20–40% of total spending is consumed in ways that do

Table 4.2. **Potential gains from critically assessing interventions**

Study	Currency[a]	Cost of obtaining one year of healthy life *		
		Current mix	Optimal mix	Improvement (%)
Malaria drug treatment in Zambia (62)		10.65	8.57	20
(cost per case cured)	US$			
Disease and injury prevention in Thailand (63)				
Cardiovascular disease prevention	BHT	300 000	2 185	99
Road traffic injury prevention (alcohol)		6 190	3 375	45
Road traffic injury prevention (helmets)		1 000	788	21
Alcohol and tobacco control in Estonia (64)				
Alcohol	EEK	2 621	893	66
Tobacco		292	247	15
Neuropsychiatric interventions in Nigeria (65)		37 835	26 337	30
Schizophrenia	NGN	210 544	67 113	68
Depression		104 586	62 095	41
Epilepsy		13 339	10 507	21
Alcohol abuse		20 134	10 677	47
Mental health-care package in Australia (66)		30 072	17 536	42
Schizophrenia	AU$	196 070	107 482	45
Affective disorder (any)		20 463	10 737	48
Anxiety disorder (any)		15 184	9 130	40
Alcohol disorder		97 932	53 412	45
Cervical cancer care and prevention (67)[b]				
High-income subregion (EurA)	I$	4 453	3 313	26
Middle-income subregion (WprB)		3 071	1 984	35
Low-income subregion (SearD)		421	355	16

[a] US$, United States dollar; BHT, Thai bhat; EEK, Estonia kroon; NGN, Nigerian naira; AUD, Australian dollar; I$, international dollar.
[b] WHO subregions (mortality strata): EurA is the countries of the European Region with very low adult and child mortality; WprB is the countries of the Western Pacific with low adult and child mortality; SearD is the countries in South-East Asia with high adult and child mortality. WHO regions are subdivided based on child and adult mortality strata: A, very low child and very low adult mortality; B, low child and low adult mortality; C, low child and high adult mortality; D, high child and high adult mortality; E, high child and very high adult mortality (http://www.who.int/choice/demography/regions). The classification has no official status and is for analytical purposes only.

little to improve people's health. The potential health gains from reinvesting these resources in better ways to improve population health are enormous.

The first step is for countries to assess the nature and causes of local inefficiencies, drawing on the above analysis. It is then necessary to assess the costs and likely impact of the possible solutions. It is possible to improve efficiency, as Lebanon has recently shown (Box 4.2). While it might not be possible for all countries to match that country's results, substantial gains can be made almost everywhere.

Incentives, health financing and efficiency

Preceding sections suggested specific actions to improve efficiency in the 10 areas identified. In this section, the focus is on the incentives – and

Table 4.3. **Potential efficiency savings by cost and country-income category**

Income category	Potential range of efficiency savings (percentage of total health spending) [a]	Potential efficiency savings per capita (US$) [b]		Potential range of efficiency savings across total population (US$ billion)	
		Mean	Range	Mean	Range
Human resources				563	110–851
High-income	8–16	492	78–629	499	79–639
Mid-income	7–14	14	7–48	61	29–206
Low-income	8–15	2	1–5	3	1–6
Medicine				115	24–193
High-income	2–3	93	14–122	95	14–124
Mid-income	2–5	5	2–16	19	9–67
Low-income	3–5	1	0–2	1	0–2
Hospitals				287	54–503
High-income	3–8	233	30–325	236	31–330
Mid-income	5–11	11	5–39	49	23–168
Low-income	4–9	1	1–3	2	1–4
Leakages				271	51–468
High-income	3–8	221	28–310	224	29–315
Mid-income	5–10	10	5–35	44	22–150
Low-income	5–10	2	1–3	2	1–4
Intervention mix				705	141–1094
High-income	10–20	602	95–774	611	96–786
Mid-income	10–20	21	10–70	89	43–299
Low-income	10–20	3	2–7	4	2–8
Total				1409	282–2188
High-income	20–40	1204	189–1548	1223	192–1573
Mid-income	20–40	42	20–140	178	86–599
Low-income	20–40	7	3–13	8	4–17

[a] Derived by multiplying a range of potential efficiency savings (human resources 15–25%; medicine 10–15%; hospitals 10–25%) by share of total health spending in the different country income groups; potential efficiency savings for leakages and intervention mix estimated directly as a percentage of health expenditure per capita (6, 69).

[b] Derived by multiplying potential efficiency savings by average health expenditure per capita [interquartile range]: 4013 [947–3871] (high-income); 139 [101–351] (middle-income); 22 [15–33] (low-income) (6, 69).

disincentives – inherent in different financing systems that can promote or compromise efficiency.

One of the key considerations is the way health service providers are paid. Payment mechanisms for hospitals and health facilities, and the doctors, nurses, physiotherapists, etc. who run them, vary substantially between systems, and many provide incentives for inefficiency. The most rudimentary payment system, as already discussed, is the health-care provider being paid by the patient at the time of need. The many disadvantages of this system – notably the financial barrier to access it places in the way of the poor and the associated levels of financial hardship it imposes on people who are forced to use services – have already been discussed at length. However, this fee-for-service payment also encourages over-servicing for the people who can afford to pay. This is another form of inefficiency.

Fee for service is a common form of payment even where funds are pooled, most commonly in insurance schemes. It is common and it is costly. Because the insurer is paying, neither the doctor nor the patient has an incentive to restrict costs and over-servicing is the inevitable result. This over-servicing often takes the form of the overuse of prescription medicines but is not limited to that. A recent study into the factors responsible for the increasing incidence of Caesarean-section deliveries provides another example. There are many determinants but both the increased demand from patients, and the increased supply by the doctors who are paid per intervention, play a role (70). Despite Caesarean-section delivery being linked to increased maternal mortality, maternal and infant morbidity and increased complications for subsequent deliveries (71–73), such deliveries increasingly take place even when natural birth presents no particular risk (74). In 69 of the 137 countries for which information is available, Caesarean-section rates are rising, costing these countries an estimated US$ 2 billion per year in unnecessary procedures (Box 4.3).

The degree to which Caesarean-section delivery is being promoted to patients by people who have a financial interest in performing them is unclear, but according to the same supply-and-demand study, where health services are provided by government, Caesarean-section rates plummet. Specifically, a doubling in the share of health spending derived from government sources was found to correspond to a 29.8% (9.6–50%) decrease in Caesarean-section rates (70).

Box 4.2. **Lebanon's reforms: improving health system efficiency, increasing coverage and lowering out-of-pocket spending**

In 1998 Lebanon spent 12.4% of its GDP on health, more than any other country in the Eastern Mediterranean Region. Out-of-pocket payments, at 60% of total health spending, were also among the highest in the region, constituting a significant obstacle to low-income people. Since then, a series of reforms has been implemented by the Ministry of Health to improve equity and efficiency.

The key components of this reform have been: a revamping of the public-sector primary-care network; improving quality in public hospitals; and improving the rational use of medical technologies and medicines. The latter has included increasing the use of quality-assured generic medicines. The Ministry of Health has also sought to strengthen its leadership and governance functions through a national regulatory authority for health and biomedical technology, an accreditation system for all hospitals, and contracting with private hospitals for specific inpatient services at specified prices. It now has a database that it uses to monitor service provision in public and private health facilities.

Improved quality of services in the public sector, at both the primary and tertiary levels, has resulted in increased utilization, particularly among the poor. Being a more significant provider of services, the Ministry of Health is now better able to negotiate rates for the services it buys from private hospitals and can use the database to track the unit costs of various hospital services.

Utilization of preventive, promotive and curative services, particularly among the poor, has improved since 1998, as have health outcomes. Reduced spending on medicines, combined with other efficiency gains, means that health spending as a share of GDP has fallen from 12.4% to 8.4%. Out-of-pocket spending as a share of total health spending fell from 60% to 44%, increasing the levels of financial risk protection.

Most systems which pay user fees from insurance funds have introduced controls on service providers to counter over-servicing. Many countries have also introduced co-payments or other forms of cost-sharing to encourage patients to consider whether they need to use a health service. But these measures can be costly to implement, require considerable capacity to monitor and fail to address the major cause of the problem – the incentives to over-service in a system based on remuneration per service provided.

One strategy to restrict over-servicing is to limit, through capitation, the amount paid to service providers. Capitation is commonly used at the primary-care level, whereby health-care providers are paid a predetermined fee to cover all the health needs of each person registered with them. Making the primary-care physician or facility, in effect, the fundholder, responsible for paying for any care they administer to their patients or for the care of those patients they refer to higher levels of the system, encourages a focus on prevention. Preventing more severe illness reduces referrals and stops them losing part of their funds. This might, however, also encourage physicians to delay referrals.

Capitation is sometimes used to pay primary-care providers or facilities for their services, independent of how secondary and tertiary care is financed. In this case, primary-care providers may well have an incentive to refer upwards early, or when patients do not really need higher-level care, as a way of protecting their budgets.

In hospitals, the equivalent of fee-for-service payments is payment according to length of stay. As with fee-for-service payments for clinical services, payment according to length of stay consistently leads to longer periods of inpatient care and, hence, higher costs than are medically necessary (76, 77).

A more efficient mechanism uses case-based payment of some sort, such as diagnostic-related groups (DRGs), where different pathologies are bundled into homogenous cost groups that are then ascribed an average treatment cost. A fixed reimbursement goes to the hospital regardless of how intensively it decides to treat patients or how long they stay there. The downside is that hospitals can discharge patients early so they can readmit them to gain an additional payment for a new DRG episode. Many countries and insurance funds – and not just those in high-income settings – have introduced some form of case-based payment in their hospital financing systems to control costs and encourage efficiency. Such countries include Kazakhstan, Kyrgyzstan, Thailand and Turkéy (78–81).

In Sweden, a comparison of local government areas (counties) that used DRG-based remuneration with those that did not suggested cost savings of about 10% (82). In

---

Box 4.3. **Global variation in recourse to Caesarean section**

The number of Caesarean sections varies enormously between countries, with richer ones and those in transition having excessive recourse to the procedure, and economically deprived countries, mainly in Africa, failing to meet demand. Data for Caesarean sections performed in 137 countries in 2007 show that in 54 countries, Caesarean births represented less than 10% of all births; in 69 countries, the percentage was more than 15%. Only 14 countries reported rates in the recommended 10–15% range.

A country-specific analysis based on WHO-CHOICE (CHOosing Interventions that are Cost Effective) methods reveals that the cost of global excess Caesarean sections is over US$ 2 billion annually. Unnecessary global Caesarean sections in 2008 outnumbered necessary ones. Because of the overwhelming concentration of excess Caesarean sections in countries with high income levels (and therefore high price levels), the cost of the global excess Caesarean sections in 2008 could have potentially financed needed procedures in poorer countries nearly 6 times over.

Source: (75).

the USA, the average length of hospital stays is reported to have fallen under DRG regimes compared with other remuneration methods (*83*). However, both capitation and DRG-based remuneration require the ability to measure costs accurately before they are implemented and to monitor their impact over time.

The alternative to remunerating health-care workers per service or by capitation is to pay fixed salaries. The challenge here is to offer incentives to people who otherwise have no financial stake in doing better. The United Kingdom's National Health Service introduced a bonus incentive scheme for general practitioners in 2004 designed to encourage them to improve care, especially in monitoring certain conditions (heart failure, asthma, diabetes). The bonus can amount to several thousand pounds a year and form a substantial part of a practitioner's income (*84*).

Several countries have begun to develop mixed-payment systems at both the hospital and individual service provider levels on the assumption that a judicious mix of payment methods can achieve greater efficiency and quality than a single-payment model (*85*). The German system, for example, combines budgets with DRG payment at hospital level with incentives to control costs. In Finland, doctors are paid through a mix of salary, capitation and fee for service.

Paying for performance

Paying for good performance is conceptually the opposite of Medicare's so-called never-events approach, rewarding doctors and nurses for getting it right rather than refusing to pay when they get it wrong. Many performance-incentive schemes have been implemented over the past few decades under a variety of labels – pay for performance, performance-based contracting, performance-based financing and results-based financing – but all boil down to rewarding the delivery of specific services to encourage higher coverage, better quality or improved health outcomes (*86*).

Some have had positive outcomes in several high-income countries in addition to the United Kingdom experience outlined previously in this chapter. In the USA there are more than 200 pay-for-performance programmes, France has a national programme, and Spain and Italy have local-level or small-scale pilot projects (*84*). Evaluations suggest that the performance-incentive schemes have improved physician and/or hospital performance against a set of measures that vary by setting but include quality indicators, such as adherence to best practices in care, controlling blood pressure levels in patients and reducing diabetes complication rates (*87, 88*). There is evidence, however, that these incentives sometimes have not resulted in improved provider performance (*89*). Even where they appear to have some impact, their cost–effectiveness has rarely been considered. Are the improved levels of performance worth the additional payments to secure them? Are there more cost-effective ways to achieve the same outcomes? These questions have not been addressed (*90*).

In recent years, this type of payment mechanism has been introduced in various forms in developing countries, often as a pilot project with donor funding, and often for child and maternal care interventions (*91*).

Such countries include Burundi, Cambodia, Cameroon, the Democratic Republic of Congo, Egypt, Haiti, India, Nicaragua and Rwanda. Improved performance has been reported in several areas of care, including the number of antenatal visits, the proportion of women delivering in a health facility and child immunization coverage (92, 93).

However, the promising results need to be regarded with caution given the limited evidence and less than robust evaluation studies, though a recent cross-country review suggested that they can be a useful tool to improve efficiency if implemented correctly (94). This requires a clear statement of the rules of the game and what is expected from each participant. It might also involve strengthening the information system and monitoring function to counter perverse incentives, where providers try to exploit the system by focusing on higher-reward procedures and patients to boost income, or neglect procedures and patients that offer lower rewards. This type of behaviour has been reported in both high- and low-income settings (95–97).

There are two further concerns about performance-incentive schemes. First, if payment for performance is introduced for different programmes separately and independently, the result may well be competitive performance incentives – each programme vying to get the providers to do their work rather than that of other programmes. Where donors are involved, recipient countries need to be making the decisions, determining how performance incentives fit in with their overall health financing and service delivery strategies, and how, where and for what, incentives should be paid.

Second, the focus on financial rewards can affect provider behaviour in more subtle ways by making individual health workers, for example, feel that their competence is being questioned or that their intrinsic desire to do a good job is unappreciated or being rejected (98). Such a focus can also encourage health workers to expect bonuses for every act performed (99).

Strategic purchasing

Paying for performance is only one of the considerations when allocating funds to ensure that good quality services are available to those who need them and that the system functions efficiently. Traditionally, providers have been reimbursed for the services they provide and/or governments allocate budgets to various levels of government, departments and programmes based largely on the funding they received the previous year. This has been termed passive purchasing (100, 101). More active purchasing can improve quality and efficiency by examining: population health needs and how they vary across the country; the interventions and services that best meet these needs and community expectations given the available resources, and the optimum mix of promotion, prevention, treatment and rehabilitation; how these interventions and services should be purchased or provided, including contractual mechanisms and provider payment systems such as those discussed earlier in this chapter; and from whom should they be purchased, taking into account the availability of providers and their levels of quality and efficiency (102).

It is not a simple choice between passive and active purchasing. Countries will decide where they can operate based on their ability to collect, monitor and interpret the necessary information, and encourage and enforce standards of quality and efficiency. Passive purchasing leads to inefficiency. Even if countries feel they do not yet have the technical and informational capacities to move rapidly towards active purchasing, they can develop a framework for doing so over time. There may well be a role for payment based on performance under active purchasing, but it is likely to work better if it is part of an overall approach that includes all the other elements.

The instruments used for strategic purchasing might need to be changed and modified over time. As already indicated, most advanced health financing systems exploit several methods of provider payment to try to achieve the right mix of incentives. Many countries have moved back and forth between them, sometimes for technical and sometimes for political reasons. This is the reality of health-care systems: policy-makers must juggle various options while engaging in broader – and often politicized – debates about the merits of various methods for paying providers and purchasing services to meet population needs.

Fragmentation

Each country needs to find pragmatic solutions for paying providers and purchasing services that reflect local conditions. Whatever choices are made, some degree of pre-payment and pooling will form the basis of health-care systems that best serve the needs of their populations. The bigger the risk pools, the better. Large pools offer several advantages, notably a greater capacity to meet the costs of occasional, costly diseases. The most efficient health systems avoid fragmentation in pooling but also in channelling funds and distributing resources. As discussed in previous chapters, fragmentation limits the scope for the cross-subsidies that are necessary in a pooling system, between rich and poor, and the healthy and sick. In the USA, fragmented pooling is perceived to be one of the reasons for the failure to reach universal coverage despite high levels of health spending (*103*).

Fragmentation can also be inefficient. Systems with multiple funding channels and pools, each with its own administrative costs, duplicate effort, are expensive to run and require coordination. Similarly, fragmentation in other parts of the system – running hospitals, distributing medicines and equipment, supporting laboratory systems – results in unnecessary waste and duplication.

Public health programmes, such as those for tuberculosis (TB) and HIV control, are often hampered by fragmented financial flows and service delivery (*104*). Where budget allocations flow from the government (often supplemented with international funds) to the programme, the programme then takes responsibility for pooling the funds and allocating them to service providers. In many cases, programmes have their own specific service-delivery arrangements, such as a TB hospital. In Kyrgyzstan, for example, the desired strategy was to have about 50% of TB patients managed by primary-care facilities, but only 3–4% of total spending on TB occurred at this level because of the way most domestic and external funds for TB were pooled separately from those in the main provider payment system and flowed predominantly to TB hospitals (*105*). These procedures have recently been modified and starting in 2011 some of these funds will be added to the more general pool of funds for health that can support primary-level care for TB patients.

Analysis of financial flows to HIV and drug-abuse programmes in Estonia also revealed unnecessary duplication. Injecting drug users were a target group for each programme, which contracted separately with NGOs skilled at outreach (*106*). In response, the government introduced a more efficient single contracting process, combining resources and packaging the interventions of both programmes (*107*).

Fragmentation is common but not restricted to the health system. A recent World Bank report suggested that there would be both efficiency and equity gains from better integrating social assistance and social insurance (including health insurance) systems in Latin American countries (*108*).

Nor is fragmentation a concern solely for national governments. There is increasing recognition in the development community that fragmented international aid delivery leads to high administrative costs for donors and recipients, unnecessary duplication and variations in policy guidance and quality standards at country level (*109*). An illustration of such duplication and waste is the high number of capacity-building seminars held each year. Often, the same people from a recipient country attend several training workshops in the course of a year, each covering similar topics, each funded by a different donor (*110*).

It is imperative, therefore, in the spirit of the Paris Declaration on Aid Effectiveness, that major donors not only commit, but act to align their efforts to promote national ownership of health plans and strategies. They can do this by reducing fragmentation in the way funds are channelled to recipient countries and by reducing duplication in the systems of training, service provision, monitoring and reporting they require. There is much to do: the number of international partnerships and global initiatives in health, each pooling and channelling funds to countries, has increased substantially since 2000 (*111*).

Redressing inequality

Improving efficiency will achieve better, more cost-effective health outcomes, but it will not be sufficient on its own. For health is more than the aggregate level of population health, neatly expressed by an indicator such as life expectancy. Health systems have multiple, sometimes competing goals: improving the overall level of health; reducing health inequalities; improving the responsiveness of the system to people's needs and expectations; and ensuring financial fairness in the way funds for health are collected (*112*). Ideally, efficiency would be measured by the system's ability to move forward on all these goals simultaneously.

At a minimum, progress in the overall level of population health and intervention coverage needs to be assessed against inequalities both within this aggregate level of coverage and in health outcomes. The substantial coverage inequalities in access to skilled health workers during child delivery and to diphtheria–tetanus–pertussis immunization within countries – taken from recent Demographic and Health Surveys in mostly low-income countries with high maternal and child mortality – were described in Chapter 1. But inequalities exist even in the richest countries, as highlighted by the recent Commission on Social Determinants of Health (*113*). A recent study in Australia suggested that patients with cardiovascular disease were much less likely to receive interventions if they were in a lower socioeconomic group. At the extreme, low socioeconomic status patients were 52% less likely than their more affluent counterparts to undergo angiography (*114*). Similar examples of inequalities in health outcomes or access to services can be found from a wide range of countries, across all income levels (*115, 116*).

Migrants are one of the few remaining groups not covered by health insurance in Costa Rica, where in many other respects, great strides have been made towards universal coverage (*117*). Indigenous populations also deserve special attention, living shorter lives, in worse health, than their non-indigenous compatriots in almost every country. A recent study reports that in seven Central and South American countries, for example, the proportion of indigenous women receiving antenatal care or giving birth at health facilities was much lower than for non-indigenous women; this inequality in coverage is one of the causes of the disparity in maternal health outcomes between the indigenous and non-indigenous populations (*118*). African-American women in the same countries also gave birth at health facilities less frequently and had poorer maternal health outcomes than other women (*118*). Different types of inequalities in access to health services exist between indigenous and non-indigenous people in high-income countries such as Australia, Canada, New Zealand and the USA, linked frequently to distance and transport costs. Whatever the reasons, health outcomes remain persistently lower for indigenous people (*119*).

Ensuring that a high proportion of the available funds for health are prepaid and pooled increases financial risk protection and access to services for all people in the population. Government subsidies derived from general revenues for people who cannot pay further increases financial risk protection and access to services. Cash transfers, vouchers and other mechanisms for reducing the financial barriers associated with transport and accommodation costs and lost work time, increase coverage further still. But redressing inequalities requires more than good health financing systems. A broader set of initiatives outside health, linked largely to socioeconomic determinants, is necessary. That said, no health system can ensure equitable coverage without the health financing mechanisms of the kind described in this report.

Conclusion

We estimate that 20–40% of all health spending is wasted through inefficiency. It is an indicative estimate, based on relatively limited data, but does highlight that there are substantial gains to be made by reducing inefficiency. Every country could do something, sometimes a great deal, to improve efficiency. The international community could also do more to improve the efficiency of the global health architecture and to support recipient countries' attempts to become more efficient.

This chapter discusses some of the most direct and practical ways to reduce waste. Policy-makers should draw on them according to their own needs, recognizing that there may be other opportunities in their own settings. Perhaps counter-intuitively, reducing inefficiency does not necessarily require reducing expenditure; inefficiency can result from insufficient, rather than too much, spending. For example, low salaries can result in health workers supplementing income with second jobs during the hours of their primary employment. Solutions need to be tailored to each country's needs, but eliminating just some of this waste would enable poor countries to move more rapidly towards universal coverage, while richer countries would be able to improve the availability and quality of the services they offer. ■

References

1. *The price of excess: identifying waste in healthcare spending.* PricewaterhouseCoopers' Health Research Institute, 2009 (http://www.pwc.com/us/en/healthcare/publications/the-price-of-excess.jhtml, accessed 7 July 2010).

2. *Where can $700 billion in waste be cut annually from the US healthcare system?* Thomson Reuters, 2009 (http://www.factsforhealthcare.com/whitepaper/HealthcareWaste.pdf, accessed 06 July 2010).

3. *The financial cost of healthcare fraud.* European Healthcare Fraud and Corruption Network, 2010 (http://www.ehfcn.org/media/documents/The-Financial-Cost-of-Healthcare-Fraud---Final-(2).pdf, accessed 2 July 2010).

4. Roses M. *Hacia un desarrollo integrado e inclusivo en América Latina y el Caribe,* 2010 (http://www.paho.org/Spanish/D/D_III_ForoPoliticaSocial_OPS_final.ppt, accessed 06 July 2010).

5. *World health statistics 2010.* Geneva, World Health Organization, 2010.

6. Chisholm D, Evans DB. *Improving health system efficiency as a means of moving towards universal coverage.* World health report 2010 background paper, no. 28 (http://www.who.int/healthsystems/topics/financing/healthreport/whr_background/en/).

7. Lu Y et al. Medicine expenditures. In: *The world medicines situation.* Geneva, World Health Organization, 2010 (http://dosei.who.int/).

8. *International drug price indicator guide.* Management Sciences for Health, 2008 (http://erc.msh.org/dmpguide, accessed 06 July 2010).

9. Cameron A et al. Medicine prices, availability, and affordability in 36 developing and middle-income countries: a secondary analysis. *Lancet*, 2009,373:240-249. doi:10.1016/S0140-6736(08)61762-6 PMID:19042012

10. *Medicine prices, availability, affordability and price components.* Health Action International, 2008 (http://www.haiweb.org/medicineprices, accessed 7 July 2010).

11. Cameron A. *Cost savings of switching consumption from originator brand medicines to generic equivalents.* World health report 2010 background paper, no. 35 (http://www.who.int/healthsystems/topics/financing/healthreport/whr_background/en/).

12. *Médicaments génériques: plus d'1 milliard d'euros d'économie en* 2009. Caisse Nationale D'Assurance Maladie, 2009 (http://www.ameli.fr/fileadmin/user_upload/documents/CP_generiques_nov_09_vdef.pdf, accessed 2 July 2010).

13. *Mémento medicament 2009.* Fédération Nationale de la Mutualité Française, 2009 (http://www.mutualite.fr/L-actualite/Kiosque/Communiques-de-presse/La-Mutualite-francaise-publie-l-edition-2009-de-son-Memento-medicament, accessed 2 July 2010).

14. Dondorp AM et al. Fake antimalarials in Southeast Asia are a major impediment to malaria control: multinational cross-sectional survey on the prevalence of fake antimalarials. *Tropical medicine & international health : TM & IH,* 2004,9:1241-1246. doi:10.1111/j.1365-3156.2004.01342.x PMID:15598255

15. *Survey of the quality of selected antimalarial medicines circulating in Madagascar, Senegal, and Uganda.* The United States Pharmacopeia and USAID, 2010 (http://www.usaid.gov/our_work/global_health/hs/publications/qamsa_report_1109.pdf, accessed 6 July 2010).

16. Cockburn R et al. The global threat of counterfeit drugs: why industry and governments must communicate the dangers. *PLoS Medicine*, 2005,2:e100- doi:10.1371/journal.pmed.0020100 PMID:15755195

17. *Production of medicines.* Geneva, World Health Organization (http://www.who.int/medicines/areas/quality_safety/quality_assurance/production, accessed 6 July 2010).

18. *Prequalification programme: a United Nations programme managed by WHO.* Geneva, World Health Organization (http://apps.who.int/prequal/default.htm, accessed 6 July 2010).

19. *Medicines use in primary care in developing and transitional countries.* Geneva, World Health Organization, 2009 (http://www.who.int/medicines/publications/who_emp_2009.3, accessed 7 July 2010).

20. *Adherence to long-term therapies: evidence for action.* Geneva, World Health Organization, 2003 (http://www.who.int/chp/knowledge/publications/adherence_full_report.pdf, accessed 7 July 2010).

21. Holloway K, Dijk E. Rational use of medicines. In: *The world medicines situation*. Geneva, World Health Organization, 2010 (http://dosei. who.int/).

22. Abegunde D. *Inefficiencies due to poor access to and irrational use of medicines to treat acute respiratory tract infections in children*. World health report 2010 background paper, no. 52 (http://www.who.int/healthsystems/topics/financing/healthreport/whr_background/en).

23. *Essential health technologies*. Geneva, World Health Organization (http://www.who.int/eht, accessed 7 July 2010).

24. *Health at a glance 2009*. Paris, Organisation for Economic Co-operation and Development, 2009.

25. Issakov A. Health care equipment: a WHO perspective. In: Van Gruting CWD, eds. *Medical devices: international perspectives on health and safety*. Amsterdam, Elsevier, 1994.

26. *Guidelines for health care equipment donations*. Geneva, World Health Organization, 2000 (http://www.who.int/selection_medicines/ emergencies/guidelines_medicine_donations/en/index.html, accessed 6 July 2010).

27. *Medical equipment in Gaza's hospitals: internal management, the Israeli blockade and foreign donations*. Cairo, World Health Organization Regional Office for the Eastern Mediterranean, 2009 (http://www.emro.who.int/Palestine/reports/monitoring/WHO_special_monitoring/gaza/Medical%20equipment%20in%20Gaza%20EB%20report(July09).pdf, accessed 6 July 2010).

28. Fisher ES et al. The implications of regional variations in Medicare spending. Part 1: the content, quality, and accessibility of care. *Annals of Internal Medicine*, 2003,138:273-287. PMID:12585825

29. Fisher ES et al. The implications of regional variations in Medicare spending. Part 2: health outcomes and satisfaction with care. *Annals of Internal Medicine*, 2003,138:288-298. PMID:12585826

30. Fisher ES. Medical care—is more always better? *The New England Journal of Medicine*, 2003,349:1665-1667. doi:10.1056/NEJMe038149 PMID:14573739

31. Maynard A. *Payment for performance (P4P): international experience and a cautionary proposal for Estonia*. Copenhagen, World Health Organization Regional Office for Europe, 2008 (Health Financing Policy Paper; http://www.euro.who.int/__data/assets/pdf_file/0009/78975/P4P_Estonia.pdf, accessed 13 July 2010).

32. Fox KAA et al. Management of acute coronary syndromes. Variations in practice and outcome; findings from the Global Registry of Acute Coronary Events (GRACE). *European Heart Journal*, 2002,23:1177-1189. doi:10.1053/euhj.2001.3081 PMID:12127920

33. Peterson S, Eriksson M, Tibblin G. Practice variation in Swedish primary care. *Scandinavian Journal of Primary Health Care*, 1997,15:68-75. doi:10.3109/02813439709018490 PMID:9232706

34. de Jong J, Groenewegen P, Westert GP. Medical practice variation: Does it cluster within general practitioners' practices? In: Westert GP, Jabaaij L, Schellevis GF, eds. *Morbidity, performance and quality in primary care. Dutch general practice on stage*. Abingdon, Radcliffe, 2006.

35. Hernandez P et al. *Measuring expenditure for the health workforce: evidence and challenges*. World health report 2006 background paper (http://www.who.int/nha/docs/Paper%20on%20HR.pdf, accessed 7 July 2010).

36. *The world health report 2006 - working together for health*. Geneva, World Health Organization, 2006.

37. Kurowski C et al. *Human resources for health: requirements and availability in the context of scaling-up priority interventions in low-income countries - case studies from Tanzania and Chad*. London, London School of Hygiene and Tropical Medicine, 2003 (HEFP working paper 01/04).

38. Sousa A et al. *Measuring the efficiency of human resources for health for attaining health outcomes across sub-national units in Brazil*. World health report 2006 background paper (http://www.who.int/hrh/documents/measuring_efficiency_Brazil.pdf, accessed 7 July 2010).

39. DeCoster C et al. Inappropriate hospital use by patients receiving care for medical conditions: targeting utilization review. *CMAJ : Canadian Medical Association journal = journal de l'Association medicale canadienne*, 1997,157:889-896. PMID:9327796

40. Posnett J. Are bigger hospitals better? In: Mckee M, Healy J, eds. *Hospitals in a changing Europe*. Buckingham, Open University Press, 2002.

41. Hollingsworth B. The measurement of efficiency and productivity of health care delivery. *Health Economics*, 2008,17:1107-1128. doi:10.1002/hec.1391 PMID:18702091

42. Zere E et al. Technical efficiency of district hospitals: evidence from Namibia using data envelopment analysis. *Cost effectiveness and resource allocation : C/E*, 2006,4:5- doi:10.1186/1478-7547-4-5 PMID:16566818

43. Lee KH, Yang SB, Choi M. The association between hospital ownership and technical efficiency in a managed care environment. *Journal of Medical Systems*, 2009,33:307-315. doi:10.1007/s10916-008-9192-2 PMID:19697697

44. Steinmann L, Zweifel P. On the (in)efficiency of Swiss hospitals. *Applied Economics*, 2003,35:361-370. doi:10.1080/00036840210167183

45. Filippini M, Farsi M. *An analysis of efficiency and productivity in Swiss hospitals*. Report to Swiss Federal Statistical Office and Swiss Federal Office for Social Security, 2004 (http://www.bfs.admin.ch/bfs/portal/de/index/themen/14/03/01/dos/01.Document.80194.pdf, accessed 7 July 2010).

46. Herr A. Cost and technical efficiency of German hospitals: does ownership matter? *Health Economics*, 2008,17:1057-1071. doi:10.1002/hec.1388 PMID:18702100

47. Staat M. Efficiency of hospitals in Germany: a DEA-bootstrap approach. *Applied Economics*, 2006,38:2255-2263. doi:10.1080/00036840500427502

48. Masiye F. Investigating health system performance: an application of data envelopment analysis to Zambian hospitals. *BMC Health Services Research*, 2007,7:58- doi:10.1186/1472-6963-7-58 PMID:17459153

49. Bates DW et al. Research Priority Setting Working Group of the WHO World Alliance for Patient SafetyGlobal priorities for patient safety research. *BMJ*, 2009,338:b1775- doi:10.1136/bmj.b1775 PMID:19443552

50. *First Global Patient Safety Challenge*. World Health Organization Alliance of Patient Safety (http://www.who.int/gpsc/country_work/burden_hcai/en/index.html, accessed 4 June 2010).

51. Kohn TL, Corrigan MJ, Donaldson SM. *To err is human: building a safer health system*. Committee on Quality of Health Care in America, Institute of Medicine. Washington, DC, National Academy Press, 1999.

52. Pronovost P et al. An intervention to decrease catheter-related bloodstream infections in the ICU. *The New England Journal of Medicine*, 2006,355:2725-2732. doi:10.1056/NEJMoa061115 PMID:17192537

53. Humphreys G. When the patient falls out of bed, who pays? *Bulletin of the World Health Organization*, 2009,87:169-170. doi:10.2471/BLT.09.030309 PMID:19377709

54. *Handbook for curbing corruption in public procurement - experiences from Indonesia, Malaysia and Pakistan*. Berlin, Transparency International, 2006.

55. Becker D, Kessler D, McClellan M. Detecting Medicare abuse. *Journal of Health Economics*, 2005,24:189-210. doi:10.1016/j.jhealeco.2004.07.002 PMID:15617794

56. Baghdadi-Sabeti G, Serhan F. *Good governance form medicines programme: an innovative approach to prevent corruption in the pharmaceutical sector*. World health report 2010 background paper, no. 25 (http://www.who.int/healthsystems/topics/financing/healthreport/whr_background/en).

57. Medicines Transparency Alliance (MeTA). (http://www.medicinestransparency.org/, accessed 6 July 2010).

58. Siddiqi S et al. Framework for assessing governance of the health system in developing countries: gateway to good governance. *Health policy (Amsterdam, Netherlands)*, 2009,90:13-25. doi:10.1016/j.healthpol.2008.08.005 PMID:18838188

59. WHO CHOICE Database. Geneva, World Health Organization, 2010 (http://www.who.int/choice, accessed 7 July 2010).

60. Disease Control Priorities Project. (http://www.dcp2.org, accessed 7 July 2010).

61. Hutubessy R, Chisholm D, Edejer TTT. Generalized cost-effectiveness analysis for national-level priority-setting in the health sector. *Cost effectiveness and resource allocation : C/E*, 2003,1:8- doi:10.1186/1478-7547-1-8 PMID:14687420

62. Chanda P et al. A cost-effectiveness analysis of artemether lumefantrine for treatment of uncomplicated malaria in Zambia. *Malaria Journal*, 2007,6:21- doi:10.1186/1475-2875-6-21 PMID:17313682

63. *Unpublished analysis from the SPICE project (Setting Priorities using Information on Cost-Effectiveness): informing policy choices and health system reform in Thailand*. Brisbane, University of Queensland, 2010 (http://www.uq.edu.au/bodce/docs/Spice_Brochure.pdf, accessed 7 July 2010).

64. Lai T et al. Costs, health effects and cost-effectiveness of alcohol and tobacco control strategies in Estonia. *Health policy (Amsterdam, Netherlands)*, 2007,84:75-88. doi:10.1016/j.healthpol.2007.02.012 PMID:17403551

65. Gureje O et al. Cost-effectiveness of an essential mental health intervention package in Nigeria. *World psychiatry : official journal of the World Psychiatric Association (WPA)*, 2007,6:42-48. PMID:17342226

66. Andrews G et al. Utilising survey data to inform public policy: comparison of the cost-effectiveness of treatment of ten mental disorders. *The British journal of psychiatry : the journal of mental science*, 2004,184:526-533. doi:10.1192/bjp.184.6.526 PMID:15172947

67. Ginsberg GM et al. Screening, prevention and treatment of cervical cancer – a global and regional generalized cost-effectiveness analysis. *Vaccine*, 2009,27:6060-6079. doi:10.1016/j.vaccine.2009.07.026 PMID:19647813

68. Hogan C et al. Medicare beneficiaries' costs of care in the last year of life. *Health Aff (Millwood)*, 2001,20:188-195. doi:10.1377/hlthaff.20.4.188 PMID:11463076

69. National Health Accounts [online database]. Geneva, World Health Organization (http://www.who.int/nha, accessed 7 July 2010).

70. Lauer JA et al. *Determinants of caesarean section rates in developed countries: supply, demand and opportunities for control*. World health report 2010 background paper, no. 29 (http://www.who.int/healthsystems/topics/financing/healthreport/whr_background/en).

71. Minkoff H, Chervenak FA. Elective primary cesarean delivery. *The New England Journal of Medicine*, 2003,348:946-950. doi:10.1056/NEJMsb022734 PMID:12621140

72. Bewley S, Cockburn JI. I. The unethics of 'request' caesarean section. *BJOG : an international journal of obstetrics and gynaecology*, 2002,109:593-596. PMID:12118633

73. Villar J et al. WHO 2005 global survey on maternal and perinatal health research groupCaesarean delivery rates and pregnancy outcomes: the 2005 WHO global survey on maternal and perinatal health in Latin America. *Lancet*, 2006,367:1819-1829. doi:10.1016/S0140-6736(06)68704-7 PMID:16753484

74. Declercq E, Menacker F, MacDorman M. Rise in "no indicated risk" primary caesareans in the United States, 1991–2001: cross sectional analysis. *BMJ (Clinical research ed.)*, 2005,330:71-72. doi:10.1136/bmj.38279.705336.0B PMID:15556953

75. Gibbons L et al. *The global numbers and costs of additionally needed and unnecessary caesarean sections performed per year: overuse as a barrier to universal coverage.* World health report 2010 background paper, no. 30 (http://www.who.int/healthsystems/topics/financing/healthreport/whr_background/en).

76. McDonagh MS, Smith DH, Goddard M. Measuring appropriate use of acute beds. A systematic review of methods and results. *Health policy (Amsterdam, Netherlands)*, 2000,53:157-184. doi:10.1016/S0168-8510(00)00117-2 PMID:10996065

77. Pileggi C et al. Inappropriate hospital use by patients needing urgent medical attention in Italy. *Public Health*, 2004,118:284-291. doi:10.1016/j.puhe.2003.06.002 PMID:15121437

78. Kutzin J et al. Bismarck meets Beveridge on the Silk Road: coordinating funding sources to create a universal health financing system in Kyrgyzstan. *Bulletin of the World Health Organization*, 2009,87:549-554. doi:10.2471/BLT.07.049544 PMID:19649370

79. Burduja D. Health services policies and case mix - what would you expect (or not) to happen? Selected findings from Romania and Turkey, 2000–2008. *BMC Health Services Research*, 2008,8:Suppl 1A5- doi:10.1186/1472-6963-8-S1-A5

80. Hirunrassamee S, Ratanawijitrasin S. Does your health care depend on how your insurer pays providers? Variation in utilization and outcomes in Thailand. *International Journal of Health Care Finance and Economics*, 2009,9:153-168. doi:10.1007/s10754-009-9062-6 PMID:19396629

81. O'Dougherty S et al. Case Based Hospital Payment System. In: Langenbrunner JC, Cashin C, O'Dougherty S, eds. *Designing and Implementing Health Care Provider Payment Systems*. Washington, DC, The World Bank, 2009.

82. Gerdtham UG et al. Internal markets and health care efficiency: a multiple-output stochastic frontier analysis. *Health Economics*, 1999,8:151-164. doi:10.1002/(SICI)1099-1050(199903)8:2<151::AID-HEC411>3.0.CO;2-Q PMID:10342728

83. Culyer A, Newhouse J. Government purchasing of health services. In: Chalkey M, Malcomson J, eds. *Handbook of health economics*. Amsterdam, Elsevier, 2010.

84. Elovainio R. *Performance incentives for health in high-income countries – key issues and lessons learned.* World health report 2010 background paper, no. 32 (http://www.who.int/healthsystems/topics/financing/healthreport/whr_background/en).

85. Park M et al. *Provider payments and cost-containment – lessons from OECD countries.* Geneva, World Health Organization, 2007 (Health Systems Financing Technical Briefs for Policy-makers, WHO/HSS/HSF/PB/07/02; http://www.who.int/health_financing/documents/pb_e_07_2-provider_payments.pdf, accessed 6 July 2010).

86. Perrot J et al. *Performance incentives for health care providers.* Geneva, World Health Organization, 2010 (Health Systems Financing Discussion Paper, HSS/HSF/DP.E.10.1; http://www.who.int/contracting/DP_10_1_EN.pdf, accessed 7 July 2010).

87. Campbell S et al. Quality of primary care in England with the introduction of pay for performance. *The New England Journal of Medicine*, 2007,357:181-190. doi:10.1056/NEJMsr065990 PMID:17625132

88. Lindenauer PK et al. Public reporting and pay for performance in hospital quality improvement. *The New England Journal of Medicine*, 2007,356:486-496. doi:10.1056/NEJMsa064964 PMID:17259444

89. Oldroyd J et al. Providing healthcare for people with chronic illness: the views of Australian GPs. *The Medical Journal of Australia*, 2003,179:30-33. PMID:12831381

90. Fleetcroft R, Cookson R. Do the incentive payments in the new NHS contract for primary care reflect likely population health gains? *Journal of Health Services Research & Policy*, 2006,11:27-31. doi:10.1258/135581906775094316 PMID:16378529

91. Eichler R, Levine R, Performance-based Incentives Working Group, eds. *Performance incentives for global health: potential and pitfalls.* Washington, DC, Center for Global Development, 2009.

92. Eichler R et al. Going to scale with a performance incentive model. In: Eichler R, Levine R, Performance-based Incentives Working Group, eds. *Performance incentives for global health.* Washington, DC, Center for Global Development, 2009.

93. Basinga P et al. *Paying primary health care centers for performance in Rwanda.* Washington, DC, The World Bank, 2010 (Policy Research Working Paper No. 5190).

94. Toonen J et al. *Learning lessons on implementing performance based financing from a multi-country evaluation.* Royal Tropical Institute in collaboration with Cordaid and the World Health Organization. Amsterdam, Royal Tropical Institute, 2009 (http://www.who.int/contracting/PBF.pdf, accessed 4 June 2010).

95. Oxman AD, Fretheim A. *An overview of research on the effects of results-based financing.* Oslo, Norwegian Knowledge Centre for Health Services, 2008.

96. Petersen LA et al. Does pay-for-performance improve the quality of health care? *Annals of Internal Medicine*, 2006,145:265-272. PMID:16908917

97. Cowley J. Effects of health worker incentive payment on safe motherhood indicators in Burundi. Presentation at STI symposium, Basel, 27 November 2008. (http://www.swisstph.ch/fileadmin/user_upload/Pdfs/STI_Symposium_08_Cowley.pdf, accessed on August 4 2010).

98. Wynia MK. The risks of rewards in health care: how pay-for-performance could threaten, or bolster, medical professionalism. *Journal of General Internal Medicine*, 2009,24:884-887. doi:10.1007/s11606-009-0984-y PMID:19387747

99. McDonald R, Roland M. Pay for performance in primary care in England and California: comparison of unintended consequences. *Annals of Family Medicine*, 2009,7:121-127. doi:10.1370/afm.946 PMID:19273866

100. Figueras J, Robinson R, Jakubowski E. Purchasing to improve health systems performance: drawing the lessons. In: Figueras J, Robinson R, Jakubowski E, eds. *Purchasing to improve health systems performance*. World Health Organization on behalf of the European Observatory for Health Systems and Policies. Maidenhead, Open University Press, 2005.

101. Kutzin J. A descriptive framework for country-level analysis of health care financing arrangements. *Health Policy*, 2001,56:171-204. doi:10.1016/S0168-8510(00)00149-4 PMID:11399345

102. Preker AS et al. *Public ends, private means. Strategic purchasing of health services: strategic purchasing of value for money in health care*. Washington, DC, The World Bank, 2007.

103. Walgate R. European health systems face scrutiny in US debate. *Lancet*, 2009,374:1407-1408. doi:10.1016/S0140-6736(09)61845-6 PMID:19866517

104. Kutzin J, Cashin C, Jakab M. *Financing of public health services and programs: time to look into the black box. Implementing health financing reform: lessons from countries in transition*. Copenhagen, World Health Organization Regional Office for Europe and the European Observatory on Health Systems and Policies, 2010.

105. Akkazieva B et al. *Review of total health expenditures on TB programme in Kyrgyzstan, 2007: NHA sub-accounts on TB control programme*. Bishkek, Health Policy Analysis Centre, 2007 (Policy Research Paper No. 55; http://pdf.usaid.gov/pdf_docs/PNADP453.pdf, accessed 7 July 2010).

106. Alban A, Kutzin J. *Scaling up treatment and care for HIV/AIDS and TB and accelerating prevention within the health system in the Baltic States (Estonia, Latvia, Lithuania). Economic, health financing and health system implications*. Copenhagen, World Health Organization Regional Office for Europe, 2007 (http://www.euro.who.int/__data/assets/pdf_file/0011/78905/E90675.pdf, accessed 2 July 2010).

107. Politi C, Torvand T. *Financing HIV/AIDS and Tuberculosis interventions in Estonia*. Copenhagen, World Health Organization Regional Office for Europe, 2007 (http://www.euro.who.int/__data/assets/pdf_file/0010/78904/E90770.pdf, accessed 7 July 2010).

108. Ferreira FHG, Robalino D. *Social Protection in Latin America: achievements and limitation*. Washington, DC, The World Bank, Latin America and the Caribbean Region, Office of the Chief Economist and Human Development Network, Social Protection and Labor Unit, 2010 (Policy Research Working Paper WPS5305; http://www-wds.worldbank.org/external/default/WDSContentServer/IW3P/IB/2010/05/10/000158349_20100510134942/Rendered/PDF/WPS5305.pdf, accessed 7 July 2010).

109. *Raising and channeling funds. Working Group 2 report*. Geneva, Taskforce on Innovative International Financing for Health Systems, 2009 . (http://www.internationalhealthpartnership.net//CMS_files/documents/working_group_2_report:_raising_and_channeling_funds_EN.pdf, accessed 2 July 2010).

110. *Reforming allowances: a win-win approach to improved service delivery, higher salaries for civil servants and saving money*. Dar es Salaam, Tanzania Policy Forum, 2009 (Technical policy brief 9; http://www.policyforum-tz.org/files/ReformingAllowances.pdf, accessed 04 June 2010).

111. Waddington C et al. *Global aid architecture and the health Millennium Development Goals. Study report 1/2009*. Oslo, Norwegian Agency for Development Cooperation, 2009 (http://www.norad.no/en/Tools+and+publications/Publications/Publication+Page?key=146674, accessed 7 July 2010).

112. *Everybody's business: strengthening health systems to improve health outcomes. WHO's Framework for Action*. Geneva, World Health Organization, 2007 (http://www.who.int/healthsystems/strategy/everybodys_business.pdf, accessed 7 July 2010).

113. *Closing the gap in a generation: Health equity through action on the social determinants of health*. A report of the WHO Commission on Social Determinants of Health. Geneva, World Health Organization, 2008.

114. Korda RJ, Clements MS, Kelman CW. Universal health care no guarantee of equity: comparison of socioeconomic inequalities in the receipt of coronary procedures in patients with acute myocardial infarction and angina. *BMC Public Health*, 2009,9:460- doi:10.1186/1471-2458-9-460 PMID:20003401

115. Huber M et al. *Quality in and equality of access to healthcare services*. European Commission Directorate-General for Employment, Social Affairs and Equal Opportunities, 2008 (http://www.euro.centre.org/data/1237457784_41597.pdf, accessed 7 July 2010).

116. Gwatkin DR et al. *Socio-economic differences in health, nutrition, and population within developing countries: an overview*. Washington, DC, The World Bank, 2007 (http://siteresources.worldbank.org/INTPAH/Resources/IndicatorsOverview.pdf, accesssed 2 July 2010).

117. Sáenz M, Bermudez JM, Acosta M. *Costa Rican health care system*. World health report 2010 background paper, no. 11. (http://www.who.int/healthsystems/topics/financing/healthreport/whr_background/en).

118. Parodi CT, Munoz S, Sanhueza A. *Acceso y gasto de salud para grupos étnicos /raciales en la región de las Américas*. World health report 2010 background paper, no. 46 (http://www.who.int/healthsystems/topics/financing/healthreport/whr_background/en).

119. Jackson Pulver LR et al. *Indigenous health: Australia, Canada, Aotearoa, New Zealand and the United States: laying claim to a future that embraces health for us all*. World health report 2010 background paper, no. 33 (http://www.who.int/healthsystems/topics/financing/healthreport/whr_background/en).

Chapter 5 | An agenda for action

5

An agenda for action

Learning from experience

No country starts from scratch in the way it finances health services. All have some form of system in place and must build on it according to their values, constraints and opportunities. This process can and should be informed by international as well as national experience. From the review of the best available evidence described in earlier chapters, it is now time to draw the main conclusions, suggesting ways countries can take action for universal coverage.

1. Pay for health in ways that do not deter access to services

The most important conclusion is that globally, **there is too much reliance on direct payments as a source of domestic revenue for health.** The obligation to pay directly for services at the moment of need – whether that payment is made on a formal or informal basis – prevents millions of people receiving health care when they need it; for those who do seek treatment, it can result in financial hardship, even impoverishment. Many countries could do more to protect these people by ensuring the bulk of domestic funding for health is derived from a form of prepayment that is then pooled to spread financial risks across the population. Prepayment and pooling not only remove the financial barriers to access, but reduce the incidence of catastrophic health spending, two key objectives in the drive towards universal coverage.

    There is strong evidence that raising funds through compulsory prepayment provides the most efficient and equitable path towards universal coverage. In the countries that have come closest to achieving universal health coverage, prepayment is the norm, organized though general taxation and/or compulsory contributions to health insurance. Neither mechanism is inherently superior, nor is there always a clear distinction between the two. Compulsory employer and employee contributions for health insurance are effectively a tax specified for health funding. That said, countries that rely heavily on employer and/or employee contributions from payroll taxes for prepaid revenue will need to consider diversifying their sources of funding as populations age – a smaller proportion of the total population will be in wage employment and contributing to the prepaid funds through payroll taxes. Many are already doing this.

    Almost every country has the capacity to raise additional funding for health, either by giving health a higher priority in government spending or by raising additional revenues from underexploited levies, as discussed in Chapter 2. Taxes on harmful

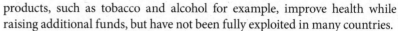

products, such as tobacco and alcohol for example, improve health while raising additional funds, but have not been fully exploited in many countries.

Contributions to the health system must be perceived as affordable and fair if the system is to be sustainable. Assessing the fairness of contributions can be complex when people contribute through various types of taxes and/or insurance. Insurance contributions, for example, might not be based on income but this could be counterbalanced by a progressive tax system overall, in which the rich contribute a higher proportion of their income than the poor. What is important is that the overall contributions are based on ability to pay.

Universality can be achieved only when governments cover the health costs of people who cannot afford to contribute. Regardless of how wealthy a country might be, some people are simply too poor to contribute through income taxes and/or insurance contributions, or are able to contribute only a small amount. With some notable exceptions, few countries where health spending from general government revenues and compulsory insurance is less than 5–6% of GDP come close to achieving universal coverage because they are unable to make sufficient provision to subsidize the poor.

Eliminating direct payments will not necessarily guarantee financial access to health services, while eliminating direct payments only in government facilities may do little to improve access or reduce financial catastrophe in some countries. Transport and accommodation costs also prevent poor people using services, as do non-financial barriers, such as restrictions on women travelling alone, the stigma attached to some medical conditions and language barriers. Many potential solutions to these problems do not fall within the realm of finance, but some do. Conditional cash transfers (CCTs), for example, have been used by the health sector in some countries to extend coverage, particularly for prevention measures, while unconditional cash transfers are typically used by ministries of finance or social security to reduce income inequalities and allow people to buy the goods and services, including health services, they need.

Difficult choices cannot be avoided on the road to universal coverage. No country can guarantee access to every health service that may promote, protect or improve health. Decisions must be made on how far to expand coverage of the population, health services and costs with the funds available. The choices countries make will be partly pragmatic – how cost-effective is a given procedure, for example – and partly based on social values that reflect a country's attitudes to social solidarity and self-reliance.

Ultimately, however, universal coverage requires a commitment to cover 100% of the population. At this point, there will still be hard choices to make, between the proportion of the health services and the proportion of their costs that can be covered by pooled funds.

2. Consolidate funding pools and adopt compulsory prepayment

It is impossible to achieve universal coverage through insurance schemes when enrolment is voluntary. Low-risk people – usually the young and healthy – will opt out, while it is difficult to ensure the self-employed make contributions. Voluntary participation might help people see the benefits of prepayment, and certainly some financial-risk protection is better than none, but in the long run, participation will need to be compulsory if 100% of the population is to be covered.

Small pools are not financially viable in the long run. Small pools are vulnerable. One high-cost illness or procedure can exhaust their reserves. Community insurance and micro-insurance have their place where it is difficult to raise and pool funds for health in other ways, and can be a useful way to encourage a sense of solidarity while promoting the benefits of prepayment. They can also offer a degree of financial-risk protection to participants, but ultimately, bigger is better, and pool consolidation needs to be part of the strategy from the outset. This applies also to small government-managed pools, such as a district health budget. In some cases, adequate coverage in poorer districts can be achieved only when there is direct subsidy from central funding pools or districts can share costs.

Multiple pools serving different population groups are inefficient because they duplicate effort and increase the cost of administration and information systems. When a health ministry and a department of social security each run health services for different population groups, for instance, the consequences of duplication and inefficiency are magnified.

Multiple pools also make it more difficult to attain equity and risk protection. Ensuring an entire population has access to similar benefits generally requires the rich and poor to pay into and be covered from the same pool. Meanwhile, financial risk protection is also enhanced when people with different incomes and health risks pay into and draw from the same pool.

Multiple pools can achieve equity and financial protection in some circumstances but this requires considerable administrative capacity. Whether these pools are organized on a non-competitive geographical basis (government funding covering the population of a province or region, for example) or on a competitive basis (multiple insurers competing for consumers), it is possible to achieve equity and financial protection if there is sufficient public funding and participation is compulsory. But for such structures to work, it is necessary to ensure *pooling across pools*, effectively creating a *virtual* single pool through risk equalization, whereby funds are transferred from insurers or regions that cover low-risk people to those that cover higher-risk people. This approach is administratively demanding, requiring an ability to monitor risks and costs effectively and to collect and transfer funds across pools.

3. Use resources more efficiently and equitably

All countries can improve efficiency, sometimes by a great deal, thereby freeing resources to ensure more rapid progress towards universal coverage. Focusing on medicines alone (improving prescribing guidance, for example, or ensuring transparency in buying and tendering) can significantly reduce spending in many countries, with no loss of quality. Other common sources of inefficiency are outlined in Chapter 4, along with suggestions to address them.

Fragmentation leads to problems in pooling resources **and inefficiencies in purchasing and service delivery.** Inflows of development assistance for health can inadvertently magnify this problem. Funding to programme-based strategies does not have to be provided through parallel funding streams, each requiring its own administrative and monitoring procedures, yet often they are organized this way.

Active or strategic purchasing of and contracting for health services helps countries move faster towards universal coverage but should not be undertaken lightly. Responsible officials for purchasing and/or contracting need to allocate resources based on value for money, performance and information on population needs. This requires good information systems and strong information management and analysis. Accurate assessment of population health needs, spending patterns and the cost–effectiveness of interventions also enhance quality and efficiency.

Incentives to provide efficient, equitable and quality services are essential whether service providers are publicly or privately owned. There is no evidence that privately owned/financed service providers are any more or less efficient than government owned/financed alternatives. From a health-financing policy perspective, deciding how best to provide services requires a pragmatic rather than an ideological approach.

Fee-for-service payment generally encourages overprovision for people who can pay (or who are covered by insurance) and underprovision for those who cannot. Beyond that general truth, payment mechanisms should be evaluated on their merits. For example, using capitation for outpatient services and forms of case-based payment, such as diagnostic-related groups, for inpatient care reduces the incentives for over-servicing encouraged by fee-for-service payment. But these approaches can create other problems, such as early discharge from hospital followed by readmission to capture an additional payment. Many countries are experimenting with a mix of payment and administrative procedures to exploit strengths and mitigate weaknesses.

Preventive and promotive interventions can be cost effective and reduce the need for subsequent treatment. Generally speaking, however, there is much greater pressure on politicians to ensure access to treatment, and many financing systems focus largely on paying for this rather than population-based forms of prevention and promotion. In addition, left to their own devices, individuals will generally underinvest in prevention. This means it is sometimes necessary for governments to fund population-based prevention and promotion activities separately from the financing system for personal services linked largely to treatment and rehabilitation.

Effective governance is the key to improving efficiency and equity. Some of the ground rules for good governance are established outside the health sector – financial management and audit, for example – but there is no reason why health should not be a trailblazer in this area. Decision-makers working in health can do a great deal to reduce leakage, for example, notably in procurement. They can improve quality in service delivery and the efficiency of the system, including through regulation and legislation.

The lessons described above, drawn from long experience in many countries, can help policy-makers decide how best to move forward, but simply adopting elements from a menu of options, or importing what has been shown to work in other settings, will not be sufficient. **Health financing strategy needs to be home-grown – pushing in the direction of universal**

coverage out of the existing terrain. It is imperative that countries develop their own capacities to analyse and understand the strengths and weaknesses of the existing system so they can adapt health-financing policies accordingly, implement them, and monitor and modify them over time.

These lessons relate mainly to the technical challenges of health-financing reform but technical work is only one component of policy development and implementation. Other actions are necessary to engender reflection and change. These are considered in the next section.

Supporting change

The health-financing decision cycle represented here (Fig. 5.1) is intended as a guide rather than a blueprint, and while the processes we envisage are represented as conceptually discrete, in reality they overlap and keep evolving.

The seven actions described here apply not only to low- and middle-income countries. High-income countries that have achieved elevated levels of financial risk protection and coverage also need to engage in continuous self-assessment to ensure the financing system continues to achieve its objectives in the face of ever-changing diagnostic and treatment practices and technologies, increasing demands and evolving fiscal constraints.

Designing and implementing health finance strategy involves continuous adaption rather than linear progress towards some notional perfection. The cycle is completed (Action 7) when a country reviews how far it has progressed towards its stated goals (Action 1), allowing it to re-evaluate its strategies and devise new plans to redress any problems. It is a process based on continual learning, the practical realities of the system feeding back into constant re-evaluation and adjustment.

Health financing systems must adapt, not just because there is always room for improvement but because the countries they serve also change: disease patterns evolve, resources ebb and flow, institutions develop or decline (Fig. 5.1).

Action 1: establishing the vision

Establishing a vision for the future based on an understanding of the present is crucial because the paths countries choose towards universal coverage will necessarily differ. The commitment to universal coverage recognizes the objectives of reducing financial barriers to access and increasing and maintaining financial risk protection. It recognizes, however, that there will be trade-offs along the way in the proportion of the population, services and costs that can be covered for any given level of resources. It is important to outline the choices a country must make. For example, in a country where most people believe individuals must take some financial responsibility for their own health, it might be decided to cover only a proportion of the total costs of services from pooled funds and ask households to contribute the remaining part directly – at least for some services. In other countries where the concept of social solidarity is strong, it might be preferable to cover a higher proportion of the total cost, even though this may mean offering a narrower range of services. Recognizing these values and allowing them to inform the overall

vision for the system is important to determining how the technical work should proceed. It can also guide decision-makers in managing the coverage trade-offs that will inevitably arise as the financing system evolves.

Action 2: situation analysis – understanding the starting point

The situation analysis should focus on the two components of universal coverage from a financing perspective: access to needed services and financial risk protection. It would identify who is covered from pooled funds, for what services and for what proportion of cost, showing the gap between what is currently being achieved and what the country would like

Fig. 5.1. **The health-financing decision process**

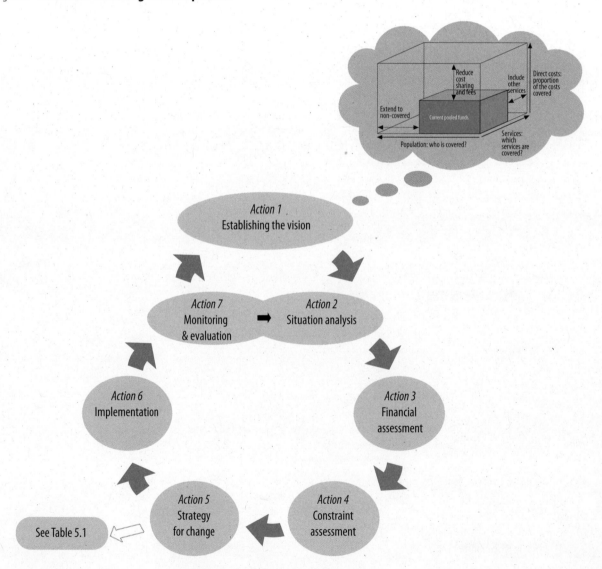

to achieve (as defined in Action 1). In planning for the future, the situation analysis needs to consider factors inside and outside the health system that may affect progress on the path to universal coverage (Box 5.1). This is not just a technical process. While it is the basis of sound strategy development, having the right information – the current incidence of financial catastrophe linked to direct payments for health services, for example – can provide an impetus for political change (1).

Action 3: financial assessment

The current and likely future availability of funds for health from government, households, the private sector, nongovernmental organizations and external partners needs to be assessed to create a comprehensive funding framework for the health system. Assessment should include analysing the share of public resources allocated to the sector over time. The lack of continuity between policy, planning and budgeting is a matter of concern in many countries. Analytical tools such as a medium-term expenditure framework – a planning and budget formulation process that sets three-year fiscal targets based on macroeconomic projections, and allocates resources to strategic priorities within these targets – can help create an overall funding picture and inform dialogue between the health and financial/planning ministries (2).

In some countries, this stage will involve dialogue with international financial institutions and external partners to assess the resources likely to be available and how they will be channelled to government and nongovernment actors. Policy-makers will also want to establish whether government spending will be restricted and how spending limits might be increased. Finally, complementary roles for different sources of funds to the health system should be considered.

Box 5.1. **Key components of a situation analysis for health financing**

Financial risk protection

- What funds are available in relation to need and what are the sources? What priority does government give to health in its spending decisions?
- How much do people have to pay out of pocket for health services (e.g. direct payments) and what is the impact of financial risk protection on financial catastrophe and impoverishment?
- Who pays what in other contributions to the health system? (This is to allow an analysis of the perceived fairness of financial contributions.)
- Who is covered from pooled funds, for what services and for what proportion of the costs?

Access to needed services

- It is difficult to measure financial access to services directly, so the analysis will generally focus on current levels of coverage for key interventions. It will then undertake an assessment of the reasons for coverage that is considered low, particularly among vulnerable groups, and the extent to which changes to the financing system would improve this access.

Efficiency

- What are the main efficiency problems in the system, their consequences and their causes?

Health system characteristics and capacities

- Systematic description and quantification of arrangements for raising and pooling funds, and using them to finance or provide services. This includes more than just tracking funds but also understanding how they flow through the system, from source to use, including external funds, noting where/how the system is fragmented and where/how policy instruments are poorly aligned. Governance arrangements also need to be looked at, notably to whom and for what are purchasing agencies responsible.
- The availability, distribution and patterns of use of health facilities (government and nongovernment), health workers (government and nongovernment) and key inputs such as medicines and technologies. The result of this assessment determines the feasibility of different approaches to increasing coverage – e.g. conditional cash transfers are unlikely to work if there are no facilities located close to the people identified as having low coverage.

Factors outside the health system

- Demographic variables, such as population-growth rates, age structure, geographical distribution and migration patterns, labour force participation, extent of informal work, etc. have implications for how fast needs will increase and the feasibility of different methods for raising revenue.
- Main disease problems and likely changes over time, with implications for the costs of extending coverage over time.
- The scope of existing social safety nets that reduce the economic impact of (long-term) illness or reduce the financial barriers of accessing services.
- Relevant aspects of public-sector administration and the legal framework, to understand how much leeway there is for changes to the financing system within the context of existing regulations and laws. Key questions include: how are health workers paid and are these arrangements linked to civil service rules? What would be required to modify them if necessary? How is decision-making on financial resources allocated across levels of government (i.e. political-administrative decentralization issues)? How are budgets drawn up in the public sector? How much scope do state bodies (e.g. public hospitals) have for redistributing funds across line items?

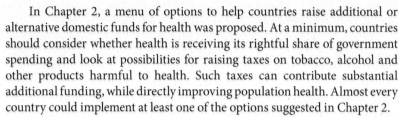

In Chapter 2, a menu of options to help countries raise additional or alternative domestic funds for health was proposed. At a minimum, countries should consider whether health is receiving its rightful share of government spending and look at possibilities for raising taxes on tobacco, alcohol and other products harmful to health. Such taxes can contribute substantial additional funding, while directly improving population health. Almost every country could implement at least one of the options suggested in Chapter 2.

Understanding the language of economists is critical to raising more funds for health. When the health ministry is seen as an efficient and prudent manager of public resources that can demonstrate progress and good results, it is more likely to win the trust and confidence of the finance and other ministries. Being able to speak the language of economists will also enhance its ability to argue for additional funding. Critical to this effort is a health ministry's capacity to draw on health policy analysis skills to produce the necessary documentation and engage in dialogue with the finance and planning ministries.

Action 4: constraint assessment

Having done the groundwork, it is important at this stage for policy-makers to identify the main supporters of change and where significant opposition is likely. An assessment of potential constraints allows decision-makers to identify policy areas that require widespread consultation, with whom it should consult and in what way. Such an assessment would culminate in the political decision to move forward.

It is in this phase that decision-makers also identify what is technically and politically feasible and determine how government can build on and support social demand for a well-functioning health system. This is a process that overlaps with subsequent actions and should be repeated regularly. What is impossible today might well be possible tomorrow. The key points to remember are:

- Achieving universal health coverage is not just a technical matter; it is an expression of a country's perception of social solidarity. The impetus for adoption is always, at least partly, political.
- Health financing systems are resistant to change, partly because any change encroaches on the interests of powerful stakeholders. In the face of countervailing forces and deeply entrenched vested interests, support for change needs to be robust and sustained from the highest levels.
- At the grass-roots level, the dynamic is often inverted. Population surveys frequently reveal a desire for change/improvement in a country's health system. Grass-roots movements for health reform and civil society groups (including consumer organizations concerned with specific conditions) can be conduits for change at both the national and international level. Communication between such groups and the health ministry helps push health on to the wider political agenda and keep it there. This has been the approach taken by the Bangladesh government, for example, in its project to revitalize and extend community health clinics. Community management groups help to support planning and management, and the interaction between health workers and the population they serve (3).

- A proactive approach to the political sphere has borne fruit in many countries. Advocacy, communication and evidence-based arguments can go a long way in eliciting the political and financial support needed to seek universality.

Action 5: develop and formalize strategies and targets for change

This is the most time-consuming and labour-intensive action. It is also the focus of most of the literature on health financing and forms the bulk of technical support given to countries, sometimes on the assumption that the other actions have been, or will be, worked through. In reality, the other actions have often been overlooked or hurried through, despite the fact they form the foundation for the technical work. The development of strategies and targets in this phase must grow out of the situation analysis and assessment of the funding context (Actions 2 and 3).

Based on the situation analysis and an accurate assessment of the likely funding scenarios, detailed technical work on strategy can begin, focusing on the three key health financing phases: raising funds; pooling them; and using them to ensure that services are available.

To illustrate the range and nature of the core decisions to be taken, Table 5.1 draws on the key messages of Chapters 1–4.

Action 6: implementation, including assessing organizational structures and rules

In this phase, some countries will need to make only small changes to maintain achievements. Others will have to instigate reform, establishing new institutions and organizations. For example, a country may decide to develop a health insurance fund as a semi-governmental authority to bypass limitations on pooling and purchasing within the public-sector financial management system. Sometimes, however, existing institutions may simply need to adapt; for example, where compulsory insurance is to be organized through the private sector. Where a compulsory insurance fund exists as a public-sector agency, new laws and regulations might be required or existing regulations reinforced or repealed.

Legislation can certainly help the development of health financing systems for universal coverage and it can also help protect an individual's right to receive health care. In several countries recently, new laws and constitutional entitlements have resulted in more people going to court to uphold their right of access to health services (4). It is too early to know the implications of this for achieving universal coverage, though researchers have found in some cases that the poor and vulnerable have benefited less from this right to legal redress than the more affluent groups who are more eloquent in expressing their needs (5).

One of the biggest challenges many countries face in this implementation phase is a lack of technical and organizational capacity. Accountants, actuaries, auditors, economists and lawyers can be essential in different settings and sometimes expertise can be scarce. It may, therefore, be necessary for countries to reassess educational/training priorities to develop the requisite skills and to develop strategies to attract and retain skilled professionals from outside the country.

The expansion of service coverage is often hampered by a dearth of health-service providers, and financing plans need to ensure an adequate supply of health workers with the appropriate skills. Financing plans must also enhance the quality and quantity of service delivery, and ensure appropriate medicines and technologies are available. Conversely, decision-makers need to be mindful of the implications for financing when reforming other areas of the health system.

Many of the changes will require intersectoral action, with health ministry staff working with other ministries.

Table 5.1.   Technical decisions required for Action 5

Principal objective	Components	Decisions
Raising sufficient funds	**Sufficiency** (this part is closely related to Action 3, and some actions will be taken concurrently)	1. Choose the mix of taxes and/or insurance contributions that households will be requested to contribute. Decide on any other mechanisms for raising revenues for health domestically – e.g. contributions from businesses. Aim to ensure a stable and predictable flow of funds into the system.
	Equity in contributions	2. Develop a mechanism to cover people who cannot afford to contribute. This can be achieved by cross-subsidization, either through general government revenues or by setting health insurance contributions higher for people who can pay to cover non-contributing members.
		3. Implement a system of household contributions that are affordable.
	Efficiency in collection	4. Improve efficiency in raising funds by ensuring the people who are supposed to contribute, do so.
	Financial sustainability	5. Make evidence-based estimations on the potential to raise funds (domestic and external) in the future and match those with estimated needs and growth in needs (linked to Action 3)
Reducing financial barriers	**Affordability and access**	6. Based on Decision 1, establish institutional and administrative arrangements to collect and pool contributions from the various sources (thereby reducing reliance on direct out-of-pocket payments in countries where they are high).
		7. Determine whether user charges have been used to provide incentives for quality, such as supplementing salaries at the primary-care level. In replacing user fees, it is important to replace not only the total funding that would have been raised, but funding for the activities previously paid for by fees. Additional funds would also be required to meet the expected increase in demand. This minimizes the possibility of unofficial replacing official payments.
		8. Determine whether there are some groups of people or some specific interventions for which demand-side actions should be taken (vouchers, cash transfers) to ensure appropriate access.
	Equity in pooling	9. Make contributions to the health system (taxes and/or insurance) compulsory as soon as possible. This will ensure that people will contribute when they are healthy, not just when they fear illness. Allowing people to opt out should be avoided because it reduces the extent to which the poor and vulnerable are covered.
		10. If there are multiple pools, reduce fragmentation by either merging them into a larger pool or by implementing a mechanism for equalizing risks across them to ensure that the people in the different pools are treated equally.
		11. Define who is eligible to obtain services through the pool(s), the services to be provided and any level of co-payments. Develop a timetable for expanding these parameters according to the financial sustainability plan described above.
	Efficiency in pooling	12. Minimize fragmentation in holding funds as far as possible.

Principal objective	Components	Decisions
Using resources wisely	**Efficiency in use of resources**	13. Design and implement provider-payment mechanisms that create incentives for increases in quality and efficiency.
		14. Because all methods of paying providers have advantages and disadvantages, develop complementary steps that encourage quality and efficiency. Important elements include tackling waste and corruption, and designing cost-effective medicine selection, procurement and supply chains (see Chapter 4 for more detail).
		15. Decide how to allocate pooled resources between different types of health services and different levels of care, while ensuring that this does not create obstacles for coordination of care across levels.
		16. Engage in strategic purchasing/contracting to ensure the highest value for money.
		17. Decide if it is necessary to develop a separate pool of funds for health promotion and prevention.
		18. Routinely monitor results and efficiency in the use of funds.
	Equity in use of resources	19. Decide how to allocate pooled resources between geographical regions, accounting for relative population size, relative income/poverty, relative health needs and unavoidable differences in the costs of delivering services (e.g. due to low population density).
		20. Determine whether there remain inequalities in coverage and health outcomes that cannot be addressed by the financing system, and that require action in the rest of the health system (e.g. distribution of health facilities or human resources) or in other sectors. Decide which other ministries and civil society organizations can best contribute to solving these problems; develop and implement joint solutions.

Action 7: monitor and evaluate

Decision-makers need to know where their country stands. Whether planning reform that will lead to a system of universal coverage, engaged in the transition or already meeting their stated goals, they need to be able to assess both their status and momentum. They need to know whether the country is moving closer to or further away from universal coverage.

Financing systems do not necessarily respond to changes as planned. It is important, therefore, to be prepared for the unexpected and be able to make rapid adjustments. To do this, decision-makers need a constant stream of accurate intelligence. In Box 5.1 we outlined the type of information needed for meaningful situation analysis, much of which relates to how available financial resources are being used. Here we turn to the assessment of outcomes, which is necessary for a country to determine whether it is moving closer to or further from universal coverage.

Monitoring needs to focus on whether people have access to needed health services and risk financial hardship in paying for them. Some of the information required for an accurate assessment is difficult to obtain. For example, while it is relatively easy to measure the proportion of people covered by a specific health insurance scheme, this is not an indicator of true coverage because we would also like to know the proportions of the needed services and the costs that are covered.

In systems characterized by a mix of public and private services, funded partly by insurance and partly from tax revenues, the picture can be complex. In theory, everyone can use government services, but in practice, people in remote areas may not have physical access to them, or may not use

Table 5.2.   **Monitoring universal coverage of protection from financial risk**

Objectives and actions	Associated indicators	Interpretation
1. Raising sufficient funds for health: what proportion of the population, services and costs is it feasible to cover?	1. Total health spending per capita	1. Must be related to population needs but the average minimum requirement across low-income countries is estimated at US$ 44 in 2009, rising to US$ 60 in 2015.
	2. Total health spending as a percentage of gross domestic product	2. This also reflects the availability of funds because total health spending/GDP generally increases with GDP per capita. Countries in the WHO South-East Asia and Western Pacific Regions have set themselves a target of 4%, although this might not be sufficient in itself. The 40 or so countries globally with GDPs per capita under US$ 1000 would not meet the minimum levels of funding needs with this spending.
	3. General government health spending as a percentage of total government spending[a]	3. Indicates government commitment to health. Sub-Saharan African countries set themselves a target of 15% of government spending to be allocated to health. In the WHO Eastern Mediterranean Region, Member States are discussing a target of 8% of government spending going to the health ministry.
	4. General government health spending as a percentage of gross domestic product	4. Indicates the capacity and will of government to shield the population from the costs of care. It is difficult to get close to universal coverage at less than 4–5% of GDP, although for many low- and middle-income countries, reaching this goal is aspirational in the short term and something to plan for in the longer run.
2. Levels of financial risk protection and coverage for vulnerable groups – a combination of who is covered and what proportion of the costs	5. Out-of-pocket spending as a percentage of total health spending, with information on which population groups are most effected	5. Empirical evidence shows that this is closely linked to the incidence of financial catastrophe and impoverishment due to out-of-pocket spending. Where out-of-pocket health payments/total health spending is lower than 15–20%, there is little financial catastrophe or impoverishment. Many countries still have higher ratios, and the countries in the WHO Western Pacific Region have set a target of 20–30%.
	6. Percentage of households suffering financial catastrophe each year by out-of-pocket health payments, with information on which population groups are most effected	6. Ideally, this would be measured directly, although indicator 5 is highly correlated with financial catastrophe.
	7. Percentage of households suffering impoverishment each year by out-of-pocket health payments, with information on which population groups are most effected	7. Same comment as with indicator 6.
3. Efficiency of resource utilization[b]	8. Median consumer price of generic medicines compared with the international reference price	8. Where this is higher than a 1:1 ratio, there is strong evidence of potential savings.
	9. Percentage of public spending on health allocated to fixed costs and salaries compared with medicines and supplies	9. This is more difficult to interpret, although most countries know when it is too high – when there are insufficient funds to buy medicines, for example. This might sometimes reflect insufficiency of funds more than inefficiency.

[a] General government health spending captures spending on health from general government revenues for all ministries, all levels of government and compulsory health insurance combined.

[b] It is difficult to establish valid, reliable and comparable indicators of health system efficiency. The two indicators are only illustrations, and countries will need to focus on other areas of inefficiency that are particularly important in their own contexts. Potential indicators include: share of total spending on primary versus hospital care; referral rate from primary to secondary level of care; use of generics versus brand-name medicines; day surgery versus hospitalizations; and overall administration costs.

them if the quality is poor or perceived to be poor. So identifying who is truly covered by publicly funded services can be difficult, even with reliable data from well-designed household surveys.

In Table 5.2 we propose indicators that have been shown consistently to be strong predictors of who is covered and the extent of the financial risk protection offered, the extent of out-of-pocket payments and their impact on financial catastrophe and impoverishment. Clearly, they do not cover every possible impact of a health financing system on people's lives. People already living in poverty, for example, will not be impoverished by health payments, but will be pushed deeper into poverty. Several other indicators, such as whether poor people have been made poorer by the need to pay for health services, are available for countries with additional monitoring capacity, but here we list a minimum set of indicators that are widely used (6–8).

We do not propose indicators for the coverage side here. Ideally, we would like to know the proportion of the population, broken down by key variables including age, sex and socioeconomic status, that does not have access to needed services because of financial barriers or other potential obstacles. This information, however, is not available in most countries and the range of services needed may vary considerably because of different disease and demographic patterns. We suggest that each country may want to monitor a different set of interventions for effective coverage. A set of possible indicators is provided annually in *World health statistics* (9), although they pertain mostly to low-income countries where communicable diseases predominate.

Regular flows of data in these areas, as well as those described for the situation analysis in Box 5.1, depend on two things:

- A functioning health information system that provides information on coverage of those in need, ideally broken down by age, sex, socioeconomic status and other indicators of vulnerability or deprivation. This requires that those responsible for managing health system administrative data have good links with national statistical agencies.
- A system for monitoring financial flows. National health accounts provide crucial information, as do intermittent household surveys, for measuring out-of-pocket spending and financial risk protection.

Policy-makers should strive to create a unified financial reporting system that is not broken down by programme, administrative decentralization or the insurance status of the population. Problems arise when donor funding for projects and programmes is tracked by parallel financial reporting systems that do not talk to each other. It is also vital to gather information from all the actors in a health system, private and public. In many countries, official health information systems collect little data from the nongovernment sector, making it difficult to obtain a full picture of the health status and usage patterns of the population.

An agenda for the international community

While countries can do a great deal for themselves by following the agenda outlined above, the international community has a vital role to play in supporting those countries requiring additional help. It is essential for development partners to:

Maintain levels of assistance or increase them to the required level

Only about half the countries reporting their official development assistance (ODA) disbursements to the Organisation for Economic Co-operation and Development (OECD) are on track to meet the targets they have committed to internationally. The other countries are falling short, some by a long way. While some donors have promised to maintain their assistance commitments for 2010 despite the global economic downturn, others have reduced or postponed their pledges. This is of great concern and it is to be hoped that development partners live up to the promises made in Paris and Accra.

Ensure that aid is more predictable

When countries cannot rely on steady funding, planning for the future becomes difficult. Some low-income countries rely on external resources to fund two thirds of their total health spending, making predictable aid flows of paramount importance. Development partners can help by structuring contribution arrangements that break out of traditional annual (ODA) commitments – as donors from the OECD's development assistance committee did in Accra, committing to three- to five-year funding cycles.

Innovate to supplement health spending for poor populations

Much has been achieved in this area, notably by the Millennium Foundation on Innovative Financing for Health, which most recently developed mechanisms for individuals to make voluntary contributions to global health when paying online for airline tickets, hotel rooms or rental cars. The sale of bonds guaranteed by donor countries, issued on international capital markets, is estimated to have raised US$ 2 billion since 2006. While such schemes have yielded promising results, much more could be done in this area. It is estimated, for example, that a global currency transaction levy could raise in excess of US$ 33 billion annually (see Chapter 2).

Support countries in their health plans rather than impose external priorities

The focus of many external partners on some high-profile programmes runs counter to the spirit of the 2003 Paris Declaration on Aid Effectiveness, which seeks to enable recipient countries to formulate and execute their own national plans according to their own priorities. What is required here is a refocusing on agreed financial contributions to national health plans, where reporting and follow-up of results take place at the national level.

Channel funds through the institutions and mechanisms crucial to universal coverage

Some recipient countries have argued that donors are unwilling to use the systems they are supposedly strengthening, preferring to establish and use parallel systems in: channelling funds to countries; buying inputs, such as medicine and equipment, and services; and monitoring results (10). One way to strengthen national systems would be to channel external funds through the recipient country's own risk pooling mechanism. This might take the form of sector-wide support, whereby donors specify that their funding is for the health sector, but allow governments to decide on its distribution across programmes and activities or through health insurance pools. Development partners should also seek to strengthen the domestic capacity of these institutions.

Support local attempts to use resources more efficiently

Reduce duplication in channelling methods and multiple application, monitoring and reporting cycles. The transaction costs they impose on countries are substantial. There were more than 400 international health missions to Viet Nam in 2009 (*11*). In Rwanda, the government has to report on more than 890 health indicators to various donors, 595 relating to HIV and malaria alone (*12*).

Set an example in efficiency by reducing duplication and fragmentation in international aid efforts

The fragmented way international aid is delivered leads to high administrative overheads for donors and recipients, unnecessary duplication and variations in policy guidance and quality standards at country level. It is imperative that major donors commit to aligning their efforts to reduce fragmentation in the way funds are channelled to and held in recipient countries. More than 140 global health initiatives are running in parallel, wasting resources and putting tremendous strain on recipient countries (*11*).

Conclusion

This is an interesting time for health finance. Two vast health-care systems, previously committed to using free-market mechanisms as the basis for funding – one in China, the other in the United States of America – are being reformed. China is moving its massive system back in the direction of universal coverage, funded partly out of general revenues. In March 2010, President Barack Obama signed into United States law a reform bill that extends health-care coverage to a projected 32 million previously uninsured Americans. While some way from embracing the principle of universality advocated in this report, the reform's easing of Medicaid eligibility thresholds extends publicly funded coverage to 20 million people who previously had none.

The reforms in China and the USA stand out, partly because of the size of systems involved, but these countries are not alone in re-evaluating their approach to funding health care. As this report has shown, health finance reform is taking place in many countries, at many levels of economic development. How each deals with the challenges faced will vary, but the programmes that come closest to meeting the needs of their populations will include some form of prepayment and pooling.

But beyond this basic truth, there is no set formula for achieving universal coverage. Country responses to the challenges will be determined partly by their own histories and the way their health financing systems have developed, and also by social preferences relating to concepts of solidarity (13). Varied as the responses may be, they will be implemented in the face of the same intractable pressures. To ignore those pressures will be to fail in one of the most important tasks of government: to provide accessible health care to all.

Every country can do something to move closer to universal coverage or maintain what it has achieved. As daunting as the task may seem, policy-makers can take heart from the fact that many countries have gone before them in the struggle to establish a system of universal coverage, and those struggles are well documented. There are lessons to be learned. One concerns the importance of social solidarity expressed through political engagement, a theme we have returned to several times in this report. It would be an oversimplification to say that reform has always resulted where there is grass-roots demand and the active involvement of civil society, but this conjunction has happened often enough to demand consideration.

In Thailand, it was one of the driving factors in the development of the universal coverage scheme that brought health care to the millions of Thais who previously faced paying out of their own pocket or forgoing treatment. Neither of these options would have worked for Narin Pintalakarn as he lay in the wreckage of his motorcycle on Saturday, 7 October 2006. Luckily for Narin, there was a third option. It depended on millions of taxpayers, a specialist trauma centre located just 65 km from where he crashed and a surgeon with many years of training. The numbers were all on Narin's side that day. And there was strength in them. ■

References

1. Knaul FM et al. [Evidence is good for your health system: policy reform to remedy catastrophic and impoverishing health spending in Mexico]. *Salud Pública de México*, 2007,49:Suppl 1S70-S87. PMID:17469400

2. *Training in medium-term expenditure framework.* Washington DC, The World Bank, 2003.

3. Uddin MJ. Health service networking through community clinics. *The New Nation, Bangladesh's Independent News Source*, 21 March 2010 (http://nation.ittefaq.com/issues/2010/03/21/all0120.htm, accessed 28 June 2010).

4. Yamin AE, Gloppen S, eds. *Litigating health rights: can courts bring more justice to health?* Cambridge, MA, Harvard University Press (unpublished).

5. Easterly W. Human rights are the wrong basis for healthcare. *Financial Times (North American Edition)*, 12 October 2009 PMID:12322402

6. Wagstaff A, van Doorslaer E. Catastrophe and impoverishment in paying for health care: with applications to Vietnam 1993–1998. *Health Economics*, 2003,12:921-934. doi:10.1002/hec.776 PMID:14601155

7. van Doorslaer E et al. Effect of payments for health care on poverty estimates in 11 countries in Asia: an analysis of household survey data. *Lancet*, 2006,368:1357-1364. doi:10.1016/S0140-6736(06)69560-3 PMID:17046468

8. McIntyre D et al. What are the economic consequences for households of illness and of paying for health care in low- and middle-income country contexts? *Social science & medicine (1982)*, 2006,62:858-865. doi:10.1016/j.socscimed.2005.07.001 PMID:16099574

9. *World health statistics 2010.* Geneva, World Health Organization, 2010.

10. Task team on health as a tracer sector. *Supporting countries health strategies more efficiently.* World health report 2010 background paper, no. 47 (http://www.who.int/healthsystems/topics/financing/healthreport/whr_background/en).

11. *Global Health: a Millennium Development Goal and a right for all.* Address by Andris Piebalgs, EU Commissioner for Development, at the Delivering the Right to Health with the Health MDGs conference, Brussels, 2 March 2010 (http://europa.eu/rapid/pressReleasesAction.do?reference=SPEECH/10/55&format=HTML&aged=0&language=EN&guiLanguage=en, accessed 28 June 2010).

12. Binagwaho A, Permanent Secretary, Rwanda Ministry of Health. Personal communication, 9 June 2010.

13. Carrin G et al. Universal coverage of health services: tailoring its implementation. *Bulletin of the World Health Organization*, 2008,86:857-863. doi:10.2471/BLT.07.049387 PMID:19030691

[INDEX]